The Greatest Pregnancy Ever

Keys to the MotherBaby Bond

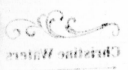

The Greatest Pregnancy Ever

Keys to the MotherBaby Bond

Laurel Wilson, IBCLC, CCCE, CLD, CLE

Tracy Wilson Peters, CCCE, CLD, CLE

The information in this book is only for general and educational uses. Nothing in this book should be regarded as medical advice, diagnosis or treatment. The information in this book is not designed to replace consultation with a healthcare provider during pregnancy nor should anything in this book be construed as medical advice. Always consult with your healthcare provider when beginning any exercise regimen or undergoing any treatment or therapy. The authors and publishers will not be liable for any direct or indirect consequences arising therefrom. The characters in this book are purely fictional. Any similarities between them and real individuals are purely coincidental.

Library of Congress Cataloging-in-Publication Data
Wilson, Laurel and Wilson Peters, Tracy.

The greatest pregnancy ever : the keys to the motherbaby bond/ Laurel Wilson and Tracy Wilson Peters. -1st ed.

2001012345
ISBN 978-0-615-57898-9

Edited by Kristen Bason and Cat Kitson
Book design by Kelly Brown and Anthony Sclavi

Dedication

Without you both, Trevor and Ryan, the seed would never have been planted. Without you Danny, the flower would never have bloomed. This book is for you, the most generous and loving of men.

~Laurel Wilson

This book is dedicated to my husband and best friend, Mark Peters. Mark has been my biggest fan and greatest source of support for more than two decades and there is no question that without his love and support this book would not be possible. Thank you Mark for working through your lunch hours and vacations so that I could realize my dreams. To my children, Hunter and Foster, who shared their mama with many families while they were growing up, and still proudly support the work that I do. You are both my greatest teachers, my greatest inspiration and I am very honored to be your mother; I love you both more than a dedication could ever say.

~Tracy Wilson Peters

Acknowledgements

Words cannot express how much it meant to us to have Robin Grille write our foreword and travel across a continent to help deliver this important message. Joe Dispenza, Bruce Lipton, and Polly Perez, we thank you for sharing your knowledge with us and believing in our message. We would like to thank our content editor Cat Kitson for all of the hours she dedicated to our book. Tremendous thanks go out to our proofing editor, Kristen Bason for helping us deliver the best manuscript possible. Thank you to Anthony Sclavi and Kelly Brown for their attention to detail and professionalism in creating the look for this book. Our deepest gratitude goes out to Polly and Eric Perez for their advice and support. We are grateful to Nealon Hightower and Barbara Harper for answering numerous questions about publishing for the first time. Tammy Archer, thank you for being our test mom and helping us stay on the right path. The CAPPA Dream Team deserves specific recognition for their ability to embrace and share the concepts in our book with open hearts. Natalie, Mandy, JoAnna, and Lisa, we are so thankful for all of the important things you did that without which we could not have finished our project on time.

From Laurel: This book grew out of a grateful heart and love that is unceasing and ever expanding for my family: my sons Trevor and Ryan, my husband Dan, my brother Harley and his family, and our parents Jane, Don, Patricia, and Marvin. The constant love you all have given me has inspired me to be better person, a better advocate, a better mother, a better wife, and a better daughter. Trevor, your birth proved to me that even profound birth trauma can be healed with love and gave me the personal knowledge for the foundation of this book. Ryan, your smiles from the moment of your birth further proved to me that a happy momma makes a happy baby. Thank you Danny, for your absolute belief in me. You are my sequoia, able to stand strong, bend and protect us all when I become a hurricane.

The depth of my love for you has not yet been located. Thank you, mom and dad. Growing up, I never once doubted that love existed in every molecule of the universe because I was so thoroughly loved by you both. Terry, you opened my mind to concepts that unnerved and excited me. Thank you for your love and for teaching me that consciousness is what it's all about. Fred Wirth, I send my gratitude to the great unknown for teaching me that babies are conscious and seeking love from conception. You changed the course of my professional life. Robin Sales, I am so grateful that you offered me the opportunity to heal my broken heart through prenatal yoga. Trish, for listening to me chatter endlessly about babies and mommas and still picking up the phone every time I ring, I love you. To the extraordinary women in my life, thank you for helping me grow into the woman who could write this book. Finally, thank you, Tracy. With you at my side, with your unwavering belief in what we are doing, we will see the world change one momma and baby at a time. Thank you for your love and even more, thank you for your faith in our concept. I am so proud of the woman you are and your willingness to be open to new ideas even when they are terrifying. Together the possibilities are endless.

From Tracy: I want to first acknowledge my husband, Mark, and my sons, Hunter and Foster. The love and support that you all give me is why I was able to accomplish writing this book. Thank you for your sacrifices along the way. Thank you to my parents and sisters for loving me and for your support. Polly Perez has been a mentor and a friend to me, showing me love and support throughout my career. Polly inspires me to never give up on a dream. I'd like to thank Janice and Barry Banther for their friendship, love and good advice over the years. I'd like to thank the entire leadership team at CAPPA, you are all so special to me and I am so grateful for your love and confidence. I'd like to thank the staff at the CAPPA office for always being available to give me opinions and support and for correcting my typos. Last but not least, Laurel. People sometimes see that our last names are the same and assume that we are sisters. I've been asked that often since we started writing the book together. I want you to know, Laurel, that you are my sister. You are such a loving person and you have enlightened me to so many things since we began working together. Thank you for helping me make the shift. I don't feel like the same person I was when we began this book and I know that you are not either. We have grown together, learned together and laughed together. I can never thank you enough for your friendship, your heart and for making me swim with stingrays (literally and figuratively).

Contents

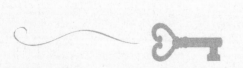

Foreword

What happens when science meets love, and for the first time the two are in perfect agreement? The result is a book such as this one by Tracy Wilson Peters, childbirth and lactation educator, doula and CEO of Childbirth and Postpartum Professional Association and Laurel Wilson, lactation consultant, childbirth and lactation educator, doula, and prenatal yoga teacher.

In a style that is full of warmth and straight-talk, this book brings mothers the most revolutionary scientific discoveries about the transformative power of their maternal love. Readers will be amazed to learn how a mother's love literally grows the child's brain and regulates their heart rhythms; in the womb, through labor, and afterwards. Only a pair of experienced and loving mothers and childbirth professionals – like Tracy and Laurel - can speak with the voice of wisdom mixed with genuine affection for parents and their babies. They tell the story from the inside. They talk the talk because they have walked the walk; there is not a patronizing word to be found in these pages.

Tracy and Laurel have rolled up their sleeves and filled this book with tons of practical help for expectant and new mothers. There are plenty of enjoyable activities for taking care of the body, mind, and spirit, with a special focus on this most important element: creating, maintaining, and surrounding oneself with emotionally supportive relationships. As a reader you will feel yourself being steered gently and capably through the potential reefs of anxiety, headaches, backaches, nausea, and other discomforts, and into a safe and pleasurable harbor. At every turn, the practical advice offered rests on the concrete footings of leading-edge science and the best knowledge gathered by two highly experienced practitioners.

In 25 years as a psychologist in private practice, I have lost count of the mothers I have spoken with who have felt utterly disempowered by their care during pregnancy and their hospital births. These women found the impersonal and coldly efficient medical approach to pregnancy and labor to be alienating, intimidating and dispassionate. What is wrong with this picture? While excelling in situations of genuine crisis, the *medical model* seems to offer little relationship to the person; it shows little concern for the developmentally critical *emotional* needs of mothers, fathers, and babies. Too often, bewildered new parents, in the midst of the most exquisite and vulnerable moment in their lives, feel pushed around, hurt, and dismissed—and finally expected to be happy that their gorgeous new baby has ten fingers and ten toes. As if all that matters is bodily survival. This is inexcusable in an era when evidence abounds for the developmentally critical emotional needs that mothers, fathers, and babies bring to labor. The rewards of a sensitively ushered pregnancy and labor can be blissful and delicious, while securing a lifetime of psychological strength and health for the babies. A revolution is warranted in how we conceive of pregnancy and childbirth: with love and attention rather than fear. It is time for pregnancy and childbirth to no longer be reduced to a medical emergency, so it can be given back to mothers. Their wonderful book is a clarion call to bring the maternal back to maternity.

It is the aim of this book to put the mother in the driver's seat, with all the support she needs at her fingertips. Mothers will feel uplifted, the importance of their role valued and elevated. The extensive and simply explained toolkit in these pages helps you to explore your feelings to know what is best for you and your family. I particularly love the fact that this book includes tips on how to interview your healthcare professionals, what questions to ask so you can decide on the right ones for you.

Your baby is a conscious person with a thinking mind, the full range of human emotion and the capacity to be in deep connection with you well before birth—this is an awe-inspiring discovery! In these pages you will be shown how to consciously communicate with your unborn child, and how to remain deeply attuned to yourself and your baby throughout pregnancy, labor, and the sublime moments of bonding that follow. You will be surprised to learn how much is known today about your unborn and newborn baby's intelligence and capacity for relationship. The most exciting news is that as you meet your baby's needs for connection, pleasure, love, and affection, you literally change her brain chemistry and neurobiology, preparing her for a lifetime of security, success, and psychological wellness. This idea is no longer the stuff of sentimentality; it is underpinned by modern brain science and mother–infant attachment research. Beautiful descriptions along the way make the book a pleasure to read and help to ground the information in your mind.

For too long, parents have been spooked by ideas about pregnancy and labor that range from the distressing to the terrifying. How can anyone relax, let go, and trust the pregnancy and birthing process after a lifetime's exposure to frightful imagery and grim warnings of overwhelming pain and trauma? It is now clear that many complications during pregnancy and in labor can be eliminated when mothers are empowered, reassured, and supported by people who are trusted and familiar, whom they feel safe with. When emotional needs are met, medical wellness is far more likely to follow. The mission these two authors have valiantly undertaken is to return this maternal and natural right to mothers. What has been taken away is now given back. The rewards of a lovingly supported pregnancy and birth are for life; they ripple into every area of human endeavor, health and social functioning—for babies as for their parents. Long may Tracy and Laurel shout their message from the rooftops!

For the delicate and intimate motherbaby bond, this book offers a unique recipe. It is a recipe for an elixir of "falling in love;" the foundation for a most wonderful start to a growing family's life together—and the best thing is: the author's suggestions are endorsed by the best of modern science. The miracle of this primal motherbaby bond is encoded as a program; it is neurologically hard-wired in both mother's and baby's brains. Tracy and Laurel take you by the hand and show you, one step at a time. They are two warm-hearted and wise mothers walking you through the most profound experience of your life. Therein lie the secrets to pleasurable and joyous pregnancy, parenting, a calmer baby, healthy brain development, and a lifetime of psychological wellness for your child.

Since modern obstetrics assumed control of pregnancy and childbirth and re-branded it as "illness," we have been lumbered with a system that too often fails to provide the empathy, warmth, attunement, and emotional safety that is the key to a smooth, life-affirming, and potentially ecstatic labor. Mothers: read on, and with Tracy and Laurel's guidance take back what has always been rightfully yours. By showing the way to a far more peaceful, loving, and emotionally healthy beginning for families, this book has the potential to change the world. It is my deepest wish that it be read by millions.

Robin Grille
Psychologist, parent educator, author of *Parenting for a Peaceful World* and *Heart to Heart Parenting.*

Notes from the Authors

We would like to welcome you to *The Greatest Pregnancy Ever*. Both of us have experienced very unique journeys along the path to writing this book. We hope the following will give you some insight as to why the concepts in this book are so important for us to share with you.

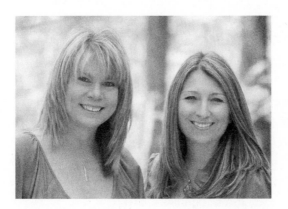

From Tracy Wilson Peters

Toni Morrison once said, "If there is a book you really want to read but it hasn't been written yet, then you must write it." For me, this is that book. I feel very strongly that this book is part of the purpose of my life. My journey to become a pregnancy and childbirth expert really started with my first pregnancy 25 years ago, when I was just 18 years old. At that time, I knew nothing about pregnancy, birth, or babies. The one thing I did know was that I wanted to be a good mother and give my child a good life, filled with love. I received a necklace that said "#1 Mom," and it was my most treasured possession. I think that even then at 18 years old, I somehow knew that what we think about, we bring about.

Despite wanting to be a great mother, I certainly made my share of mistakes along the way. I have always said that my son Hunter and I really grew up together. Even though I became a mother at such a young age, I have thankfully managed to raise two incredible sons, Hunter and Foster (eight years apart), who have both grown up to be loving, intelligent, and compassionate people.

What would I do differently? Don't we all occasionally wish we had a time machine so that we could go back and do things a little bit differently? There are a few things I do wish I could go back and change; wishing my pregnancy would go by faster, not treasuring every single movement I felt my babies make inside me, not reading just one more book at bed time when asked, and working so many hours. These are all typical mommy regrets. The thing I wish I could change the most, though, is *what I did not know at the time.*

I wish that I had known then about the consciousness of our babies (even in utero), and how much they are absorbing from us from the moment their lives begin. None of us can go back and change our past, and none of us are responsible for what we did not know at the time. This book is really my gift to all future mothers, fathers, babies, and all families.

I want to give *you* what *I* did not know; I want you to know that *you* have the power to shape a human being's life. You have the power to change your child's world and make it a better place by the choices that you make in each and every moment. Your choices affect your baby, they affect you as a woman, and they affect your family. Everything you do matters. In every mundane moment there are hidden opportunities to create love in your life. These opportunities begin in your consciousness. The opportunity to create love is always available *in the present moment* and comes from your own self-awareness. When you become fully aware of the power you have to create life, love life, and teach your children to let go and love, then you will have *The Greatest Pregnancy Ever.*

From Laurel Wilson
This project, for me, has been a long time coming. Since the very first quickening in my belly with my first child, I knew with every

cell of my body that my child was connected to me beyond the umbilical cord. I intuitively felt that my world was shaping his world, and I desired to create a world into which this child would feel welcomed. I was very young, scared, and not ready to be a mother. The early weeks of pregnancy were a roller coaster of emotions. I struggled between feeling a deep bond with the child growing inside me, and a sense of panic that somehow I would do the wrong thing, eat the wrong food, do something to cause irreparable harm to my baby. I was functioning in a heightened state of anxiety and fear, which stemmed from only wanting and wishing for the best for my baby.

At that time, I did not know that wanting and loving my child would have the most significant impact on the healthy development of my child, or that my state of mind would lay the foundation for who he would become. I did not know that addressing my fears would have been better than all of the coffee I passed by, all of the fresh fruit I ate, and all of the stretching and swimming I did to have a healthy pregnancy. Even though I was not aware of the importance of stress reduction and dealing with my fears, I did intuitively know that forming a relationship with my child did not start at his birth. It was happening every moment during my pregnancy, with the division of every cell, with every flutter of his limbs, and with every thought I had. The challenging moments of his birth and what followed were eased by the knowledge that this little person already knew me and was grounded in the depth of my love for him.

With my next pregnancy, my awareness of the motherbaby bond deepened. Though my stress levels and fears increased, I still knew that what mattered most was my relationship to this child. My pregnancies, births, and breastfeeding experiences with my sons, Trevor and Ryan, led me on my path of discovery as a childbirth and breastfeeding professional. At first it was means of healing myself, and later it became a means of spiritual awakening and service to my community. This work has challenged and rewarded me nearly every day. It has led me to a greater awareness of the emotional life of the mother and child, and has deepened my respect for life and the universal laws that support this life I live.

Unfortunately, our society tends to value things that are truly inconsequential in the great scope of humanity. We are a society that honors hard work, money, the acquisition of material objects, and the ability to multitask. While these values are not "bad," they allow us to misdirect our attention, changing focus from what really matters to the human being to the ideals of the ego. The famous leadership consultant and teacher Steven Covey said, "We are not human beings on a spiritual journey. We are spiritual beings on a human journey." Today there is a lack of human connection during pregnancy; a societal lack of honoring this sacred and integral period. How we come into existence matters. How we are conceived, what our parents think, and how our parents love themselves and one another *matters*.

Merriam-Webster defines consciousness as "the quality or state of being aware especially of something within oneself." Our culture is in a state of unconsciousness; our internal awareness is dulled. We no longer trust our instincts for pregnancy and motherhood. Families seek 4D ultrasound, consult with machines and lab tests, and compare their own experience with strangers on television. The beautiful stillness of our beginnings has been lost; the peacefulness that invites a women to place a hand over her belly and know, really know in every cell in her body, that this being inside her is beauty personified has somehow been lost in the shuffle.

The exquisite beauty of parenthood is the story being told with each and every pregnancy and birth and in every moment that a baby finds her entire world at her mother's breast. We have the ability and the responsibility to create peace in these moments. I wish to share the information in this book so that a shift can take place in our societal expectations of pregnancy and mothering. I want you to experience how spirit and science combine to make us who we are. I invite you now on this journey with Tracy and me.

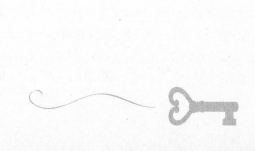

Introduction: The Disconnect

This book is not about what to expect when expecting a child. This book is not about natural childbirth or when it is the best time to get an epidural. Nor is this book about the use of medical procedures and technology in labor.

This book IS about transforming you and your baby's lives through conscious thought and awareness. It is about setting your intentions for your pregnancy and parenting, being present and creating a way of life that will transform you, your baby, all of your relationships, and ultimately the world in which we live.

This book is designed to help you focus on what matters; the motherbaby bond. Each part of the book hones in on one critical period and essential concept of the motherbaby bond and illustrates the unique and groundbreaking concepts via "keys" to help you unlock the mysteries around the motherbaby bond. The motherbaby BOND is formed via "B"e-ing, "O"bserving, "N"ourishing and "D"eciding. Be-ing focuses in on the beginning of your journey towards motherhood. Observing centers around the first trimester. Nourishing shares important information about the second trimester. Deciding gives you new insights into the third trimester. Together, these concepts are designed to help strengthen the motherbaby bond and result in happier, healthier pregnancies and babies.

Today, we live in a society where we are inundated with information about how we should have our babies and start our families. We are told from the moment we conceive which sticks we should pee on, which doctor we can see, how much weight we should gain, what we can and can't eat and drink, where to register for baby supplies, where we should give birth, whether to hire a doula (or a midwife or an OB), whether to breastfeed or bottle feed, even the day our baby will be born. Information assaults us everywhere. We are endlessly tweeted, facebooked, and you tubed about our pregnancies. From television and magazines to billboards, even in the free product samples that show up at our doorstep, everyone has an opinion about how we should experience our pregnancy and birth.

Hannah's Story

Let's imagine Hannah. Hannah has missed her period, her breasts hurt, and she is feeling very emotional. She suspects that she might be pregnant as she remembers those three glasses of wine and the samba dancing with her hubby last month. To confirm her suspicion, Hannah goes to the drugstore, stands in front of the feminine product aisle and sees eight types of pregnancy tests. Each package has multiple urine testing sticks inside, just in case the first test is wrong. All of the boxes claim she can expect accuracy, a quick response, and certain results. She winds up buying five tests because she feels so confused. At home, Hannah pees on ten test sticks. All display various plus signs, yes signs and even a digital read-out that indicate, yes, she *might* be pregnant. Hannah updates her facebook status with "OMG, it's positive!!!!" However, Hannah is still not sure she is pregnant because she thinks only a doctor can confirm that information.

That night she shares the good news with her husband, Nathan. He immediately suggests that they log on to their healthcare plan's website to search for the closest approved obstetrician. While Nathan searches the database for doctors, Hannah checks her facebook status. A list of 37 responses show up, telling her which OB is the best, where she needs to take prenatal yoga classes, giving links to baby websites, and suggesting remedies for morning sickness. She notices the sidebar of her facebook page is now covered in pregnancy-related advertisements. By the time Hannah logs off, Nathan has made an appointment with a doctor conveniently located near her office. It took exactly ten minutes for Nathan to choose her doctor.

In the weeks that follow, Hannah visits several pregnancy-related websites. They all have varying information, but consistently share information on ectopic pregnancy, rubella, risks of sexually transmitted diseases and miscarriage, foods she should not eat, warnings about hot tubs, alcohol, tooth and gum disease, anemia, the need for screenings, and even when she can have sex. Hannah finds one website she decides to bookmark. This particular website shares information on what is happening week by week during her pregnancy. Hannah immediately looks at week five and is surprised to learn that her baby's brain and heart are already developing. She feels a moment of deep connection to her baby and then remembers that she needs to check her email for work.

Hannah is getting excited. Between bouts of nausea, she decides that it is time to get some books on pregnancy. She buys a book at the local bookstore and then walks next door to the coffee shop to have a drink and read a bit before she has to go back to work. She buys her coffee, sits down, and learns quickly from her new book that not only should she not drink her double espresso, but there is really nothing on the menu she is allowed to have. Not only that, she realizes she can no longer take care of her cat's litter or eat sushi, her favorite meal. She feels deflated and realizes that her coffee shop trips are to become a distant memory.

Finally the day arrives for her first OB appointment. Hannah is nervous but anxious to discuss remedies for her morning sickness and address the list of questions in her purse. Hannah sits in the waiting room, flipping though parenting magazines that advertise infant formula and pacifiers. The nurse greets her and asks her to step on a scale while she takes her temperature. After recording her weight, Hannah is given a sharpie and urine sample cup and told to fill it, label it, and place it in the window. After completing her task, Hannah sits in a chair and has several tubes of blood drawn. Hannah is escorted to exam room B, a cold room with brochures on the wall telling her about all the perils of pregnancy, breast cancer, and sexually transmitted diseases. The nurse hands Hannah a paper gown while asking about the dates of her last menstrual period and other health-related questions. She is told to undress and wait for the doctor. As she unfolds the paper gown, Hannah tries to figure out whether to leave her belly or her backside bare. Hannah tweets on her phone, "Where's the doc, I am freezing in here," while trying to ignore her nausea.

Thirty minutes later, Dr. Smith arrives and asks her all of the same questions, while avoiding eye contact. He then asks if she has any questions for him. Hannah does not know where to start and ignores the list of questions in her purse, simply saying, "no." He tells her to lay back and put her feet in the stirrups and begins a thorough pelvic exam. Hannah stares at the ceiling, heart racing, and begins to wonder if having a baby was such a great idea after all.

He smiles and comments that everything looks great as he snaps the gloves off his hands. He tells her once the blood tests confirm that she's pregnant, they will make another appointment for an ultrasound. Hannah doesn't know why, but she feels a little lost.

In the weeks that follow, Hannah experiences her pregnancy with conflicting emotions. She begins to feel deceived by the reality of pregnancy. Her dream was that this was going to be a time of celebration, connection with Nathan, and excitement about planning their family. Instead all of her energy is focused on the drudgery of eating "right," memorizing all the bathrooms within a five-mile radius, trying to get through the workdays that used to fly by, and finding clothes that still fit. She has not had sex with Nathan since she found out she was pregnant, and they spend less and less time doing things they love. She can't mountain bike with him but doesn't want to ask him to stay home, and their wine and samba nights are a distant memory. Hannah wants to spend time focusing on her baby but she feels so nauseous and exhausted that she hasn't been able to find the time. To cheer herself up, she decides to take the prenatal yoga class suggested by a few friends.

Her first yoga class begins with disaster. After running late from work, she finds that none of her workout clothes fit. She winds up wearing Nathan's workout pants, six inches too long, crying the entire way to class. Once at class, she begins to calm down in the dimly lit room with the sounds of peaceful music playing in the background. The yoga teacher welcomes her with a bright smile, eye contact, and a gentle touch. For the first time, Hannah realizes that this was the connection she had hoped to have with her doctor.

She rests on her mat and the instructor begins to lead them through a relaxation exercise. The sound of her voice brings Hannah back to times gone by when her mother would read to her at night. The feeling that emerges from this memory is very soothing to Hannah. Hannah realizes that she deeply yearns for a bond with her baby that she has not yet felt. Hot tears run down her face and immense relief comes from this realization. The rest of class flies by and she experiences a joy she has not felt in many weeks. As class ends, the instructor joins Hannah and asks her how she is. Hannah briefly shares some of her experiences of the past few weeks, feeling lighter and lighter by the moment, grateful to be able to share. Hannah sleeps deeply that night and dreams about her baby's face.

The next day Hannah feels better. She has decided to use this burst of energy to get registered for their childbirth classes. She thinks about signing up but she really does not want to spend six weeks in class. She facebooks, "Need a birthing class, any recs?" Within the hour she has multiple responses suggesting that she take an express class at the hospital, just get an epidural, or avoid classes all together. She also is terrified by a link to a YouTube video on having a baby. She really does not have time to take classes, so she decides on the six-hour express hospital class. How hard can labor really be? She is getting an epidural, after all.

Hannah's story is one that is played out every day. Hannah is fed messages about what her pregnancy should look like, feel like, and be like by the media, her care providers, and the people around her. Hannah is told what to expect and as she adapts to those expectations, her environment begins to change her belief systems.

Hannah certainly does not want to follow these influences blindly. However, she is in a vulnerable hormonal state of pregnancy where outside influence has a significant impact. She wants to be prepared and a common rite of passage for this preparation is a childbirth class. What Hannah and most couples don't know is that for most parents, taking a typical childbirth class fails to truly prepare a couple for the upcoming birth and parenting experience. As childbirth educators ourselves, we were disheartened to learn that studies show less than ten percent of parents feel their childbirth class was the most important source of pregnancy and birth-related information.

The typical childbirth class covers the following topics:

- Anatomy and Physiology
- Discomforts of Pregnancy
- Warning Signs
- Relaxation and Breathing
- The Stages of Labor
- Labor/Medical Interventions
- Pain Management
- Cesarean Birth
- Postpartum Issues

These points focus mainly on hospital routine, anatomy, and medical procedures. Unfortunately, these topics rarely address the true needs of the family as a whole, and even worse, the research shows they sometimes leave the family in a state fear and anxiety.

The agenda of many classes is influenced by the hospital policies and routines, healthcare provider preferences, belief systems of the educators, and other class members. The typical childbirth class curriculum is often based on the facility/instructor requirements and does not address the emotional needs of the mother and her partner or the conscious awareness of the baby. That's right, revolutionary new research is proving that babies are conscious from early pregnancy.

Babies are conscious and aware in utero. The mother's environment, thoughts, and feelings determine how the child develops. It's not that the information in childbirth classes is incorrect, or even that they should not be attended; it is simply that most classes do not address the essential role of consciousness in preparation for a positive and peaceful pregnancy and birth. Childbirth classes can and do serve a purpose; however, many do not teach the most important information: that of conscious awareness. What today's families need is the opportunity to connect within, which results in deeper intimacy, awareness, and consciousness.

Another popular way that today's parents educate themselves is via the internet. As we write this book, an internet search on the word pregnancy brings up 300 million results and childbirth brings up nearly 28 million. This makes it virtually impossible for parents to filter out what they need to know. Let's be clear, this means there are over 300 million potential influences on the expectant family's psyche. It's mind-boggling. What does the internet teach us about our connection to our baby? Very little.

What's missing?

Parents don't need to be taught what to expect. They should have the ability to decide what they want their own experience to look like and even more important, what they want their experience to feel like. What parents expect becomes what parents think about. What parents think about becomes what they experience. What they experience becomes their reality and the reality of their newborn. What we think about, we bring about.

Keep your thoughts positive because your thoughts become your words. Keep your words positive because your words become your behaviors. Keep your behaviors positive because your behaviors become your habits. Keep your habits positive because your habits become your values. Keep your values positive because your values become your destiny.

—Gandhi

Part One

The Beginning

B-O-N-D

B stands for Be-ing

"What lies before us and what lies behind us is but a small matter compared to what lies within us."

—Ralph Waldo Emerson

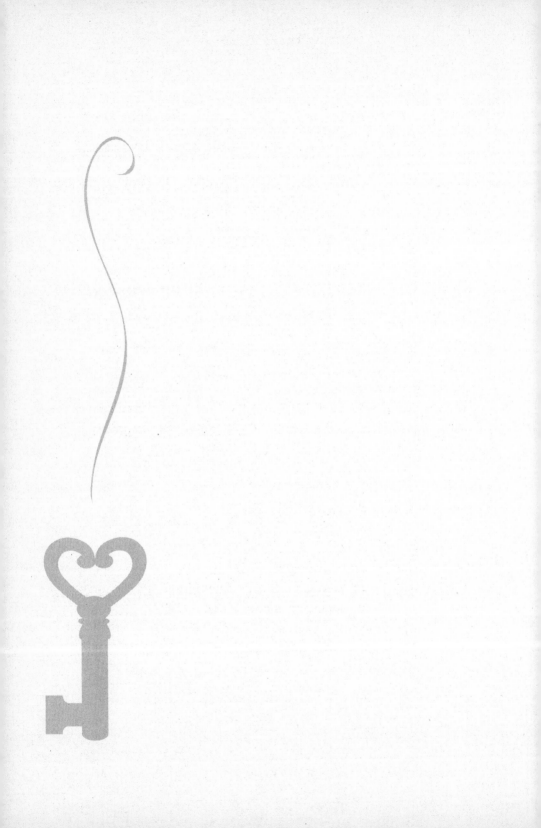

Chapter One

What is Be-ing?

"Before you were conceived I wanted you. Before you were born I loved you. Before you were here an hour I would die for you. This is the miracle of life."
—Maureen Hawkins

Every mother wants to have *the greatest pregnancy ever*, and every mother and baby deserve to have this. However, there is more to achieving *the greatest pregnancy ever* than just understanding the physical development of your baby, the reasons for certain medical procedures and tests, and the changes in your body. This chapter will introduce you to crucial information that will help you make the most of your pregnancy. This information is based on groundbreaking new science, which has previously not been available in most pregnancy books. This book shares little-known facts that can change the entire experience of pregnancy and parenting for families.

- Reducing stress in pregnancy can positively affect your baby's development, emotional and mental health, disposition and personality, as well as her overall health.
- Being conscious and aware of your thoughts, feelings, and beliefs can be beneficial to the health of your baby and your pregnancy (it can even improve your fertility).

- At no other time in the life of your child do you have more power to influence who your child will be, both emotionally and physically, than during pregnancy and the first years of her life.

This book won't tell you what to expect with your pregnancy. You have the opportunity to manifest your own greatest pregnancy ever with every thought you think, feeling you feel, and action you take. All of the relationships you have during your pregnancy are important. However, the most important relationship you will ever have as a parent is the relationship with yourself. This is the foundation for having a happy child, a happy family, and a happy life. You are important. You are literally the world in which your baby will be formed. This is an enormous responsibility, but also a once-in-a-lifetime opportunity. This book offers you a gift — the gift of becoming conscious and aware in every moment. You have the power to choose how you think, how you react, and more importantly how you FEEL. You can empower yourself to have *the greatest pregnancy ever* through a conscious pregnancy.

Becoming a parent is a momentous experience that will impact you, your baby, and countless future generations. Every pregnancy transforms the human race. Every individual who is born will change the world in some capacity. The decision to have a baby is a decision to make with an open heart and mind. Will you make the most important leap of your life? Will you make the decision to be responsible for ALL of your choices—your health, your mental attitude, your relationships, your pregnancy? Are you willing? If so, you can experience *the greatest pregnancy ever.*

When you understand the magnitude of this task, there is no other option but to wake up and become more aware. The information presented in this book is not meant to induce guilt, but instead to empower you to make changes that are right for you and your baby from this moment forward. You are not just a vessel carrying this baby. You are your child's world.

Learning how to move into a state of be-ing, or consciousness, will have a profound effect on your life and your family. Be-ing is the very foundation for the most important relationship of all, the relationship between you and your source. Your source is how you define your reason for being here, as well as how you define your relationship with every single thing in your world. This is different for every individual, whether you believe in God, a higher power, or simply that you have a unique purpose for being here in this life.

Pregnancy is a time of deep reflection, a time to look at who you have been, who you are, and who you want to be. You *will* experience a shift; your life *will* change as you know it. This journey *will* transform you.

> *Making the decision to have a child—it is momentous. It is to decide forever to have your heart go walking around outside your body.*
> —Elizabeth Stone

More than likely, you are either considering having a baby or you have already become pregnant. If you are thinking about conceiving a child or trying to conceive, now is the time to do the personal work that will enable you to have *the greatest pregnancy ever*. You have a unique opportunity here and now to become the parent you want to be before your baby is created. Even if you are already pregnant and just finding this book now, you too have an incredible capacity to transform your life and the life of your baby. Regardless of when you learn this information, it can be applied to make you and your child's life better.

What is Be-ing?

The literal definition of consciousness is the state of being awake and aware of one's surroundings. What does awake and aware really mean? The definition of consciousness for *The Greatest Pregnancy Ever* is: the act of being fully aware and fully present in your thoughts, feelings, and actions. It means being in a state of mindfulness, where you are observing the world around you. You are tuned in to your thoughts and feelings, but not necessarily allowing them to drive your actions.

What is the difference between being in a conscious state and being in a state of subconscious awareness? Scientists have found that most people's daily actions are dictated by their subconscious mind over ninety percent of the time. For example, how many times have you driven your car down a familiar road, towards a familiar destination, and realized as you arrived at your destination that you have no recollection of how you got there? That is because your subconscious mind has memorized the details and past events of your life. Your subconscious mind allows you to operate on autopilot most of the time.

This autopilot has an important role; it allows you to function without having to use up too much brain power to simply get through the day. You don't have to spend too much energy figuring out the best way to get dressed, or to make your breakfast, or to interact with the familiar people in your life. Your subconscious mind helps you move through the world in a safe and comfortable manner. This allows your conscious mind to have more energy to process new experiences. The problem is that your subconscious mind starts to create habits out of everything you do. You become less and less likely to fully experience anything new. You are a creature of habit. It's your very nature.

These habits create an illusion of safety all around you. You react to life's events according to all of the memories your subconscious mind has stored, whether these memories are in your best interest or not. For example, if you had a frightening experience with a dog as a child, your mind has stored the memory that dogs are dangerous and your subconscious creates ways for you to avoid dogs and to react as though any dog you see is a threat. Your mind is protecting you based on your past experience, even if it's not necessarily accurate. Is every dog a threat? No, but the subconscious mind might think they are. The mere act of living causes most of us to become less conscious, as we operate more and more on autopilot as we age.

So what's a human to do?

Be-ing is actually a choice that you make in every moment of every day. When you move into a state of consciousness you become aware of everything around you. You become tuned in to your thoughts and your feelings. This is called being mindful. Initially, the more tuned in you become, the more you begin to realize that the thoughts and feelings you are experiencing may not be an accurate portrayal of the present moment. Instead, the thoughts and feelings you experience are a direct reflection of your past experiences. You constantly apply your history to your present, like watching a movie over and over again. You cannot change the movie until you are aware that you have been watching the same movie over and over and want to change the channel. This realization is the first step to be-ing.

Be–ing is listening to your thoughts and asking yourself: Where did that thought come from? How does it make me feel? Is my current emotional state causing these thoughts? Is my reaction realistic based on what is actually happening?

As you become aware of the power of your thoughts, which is the true power of be-ing, you begin to realize that you actually can create change in your life. You can choose to turn off the autopilot and start to drive the car yourself. Imagine where you might go.

What happens when we are not practicing be-ing?

When you are not practicing consciousness you are unaware of your behavior, actions, thoughts, and habits. As previously stated, most people spend the majority of their lives in this state of unconsciousness. What's the problem with this? It limits your ability to create change in your life and be fully present. Dr. Wayne Dyer, a world-renowned spiritual teacher, says that what is true for us in the morning of our lives isn't true in the afternoon of our lives. If you do not practice be-ing, you aren't aware of how your reality can change. Each new day, and each new relationship you develop, presents opportunities to create positive change in your life.

You may be wondering what this has to do with having a great pregnancy. The simple answer is: *everything*. Old ideas have led us to believe that babies are at the mercy of their genes and biology. We thought that pregnancy was based on biology, and children were the products of the parent's DNA. Emerging science has discovered that while biology does indeed have a role to play in conception and the development of babies, it is not the only thing that matters. While every child will have a specific genetic blueprint, known as DNA, research has found that internal environments (thoughts, feelings, beliefs) and external environments (food you eat, air you breathe, chemicals you are exposed to, etc.) can actually change the reading of your baby's blueprint during pregnancy. It turns out that your choices can affect the way your baby's body and mind will grow. You are a baby architect, how exciting!

Here is an example: pregnancy and your growing baby are like the musicians and the instruments in an orchestra. Every orchestra has unique instruments and musicians, but you, the mother, are the conductor. You are writing your own symphony, you choose the notes and the melody. If there is something out of tune, you can change the music. You create the harmony. You are the maestro.

When you choose to conceive your baby in a trusting, loving, peaceful state, she is formed in love. This process of choosing to be conscious and aware leads you to become an active participant in your life. What you think about, you bring about. This is a critical concept in understanding the health of your pregnancy and the health and happiness of your future child.

You are often unconscious of your reactions to people, events, and places, but your body is still affected by those reactions. Unfortunately, many mothers live in a constant state of stress. During chronic stress, the body is constantly producing stress hormones, which can affect your fertility, your pregnancy, and your baby. Every experience you have is recorded in your mind in your subconscious. These memories actually trigger your brain to release certain hormones when you have a new experience. The mind responds to situations just as it did in the past. If a past experience caused stress or anxiety, the brain creates the hormones for anxiety or stress, even if the current situation may not really be cause for anxiety. Your subconscious mind believes it knows better than your conscious mind. This can create a cycle of chronic stress. Once you become aware of this cycle you have the ability to change it.

Chronic stress is one of the leading causes of illness in pregnancy, preterm delivery, and challenges with a newborn baby. Below are just a few things that stress does to a body preparing for pregnancy:

- Reduces supportive pregnancy hormones
- Increases stress hormones
- Reduces ovulation and interest in sexual activity
- Affect and even prevent the implantation of a fertilized egg
- Reduces overall egg quality
- Delays the release of eggs

Fortunately, this book will help you learn how to deal with stress: by being more conscious of your life, taking control, and using stress-releasing techniques. Isn't it time to think about what you are thinking about?

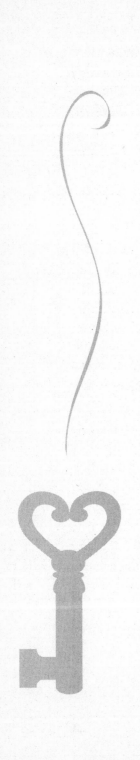

Chapter Two

Keys to a Positive Mental Attitude

"The state of your life is nothing more than a reflection of the state of your mind."
—Dr. Wayne Dyer

Is the glass half full or is the glass half empty? This question is one you have heard a million times but it is asked for a reason; it is central to your happiness and your baby's happiness. How you answer that question is critical to your fertility, your pregnancy, and your baby because it is a reflection of your mental attitude. Your mental attitude is your *perception of your world*, and this perception matters to your life and to the life of your baby. How you view your world determines your body's reaction to the world. Negative attitudes create stress in the body, and stress reduces fertility. In fact, studies show that the less satisfied women are with life in general, the less fertile they are. Additionally, happiness is related to higher fertility rates and lack of happiness is related to lower fertility rates.

In every moment of your life you judge what is happening to you. Are you more likely to interpret things as positive or negative? Remember, the thoughts entering your mind are preprogrammed from your past experiences, and those thoughts reflect your memories instead of the present situation. How many times have you heard yourself thinking or saying, "Why does this always happen to me?" or "Life is just not fair."

Sound familiar?

It's all too familiar for most people. Why? Fact: the human subconscious mind is programmed during pregnancy and early infancy by the emotional states and stress level of the mother. Your subconscious mind is what influences your thoughts and actions the majority of the time. Every single thought you now have is a direct result of how your brain developed in the womb and your first years of life, based on how your mind was programmed to perceive the world. This perception was in fact the perception your mother had of the world.

Until now, babies were seen as separate from the mother during pregnancy. It was believed that the baby's only connection to her mother was via the umbilical cord, sharing mainly nutrients and blood supply. Your baby is not living in a world separate from you; quite the opposite is true. Your baby's world IS your world. You are intimately connected, sharing thoughts, feelings, tastes, sounds, and chemical messages. Imagine the mother as the computer, filled with data, files, memory, and software. The baby can be seen as a flash drive, which connects for a short time to the computer to download all of the important data. Once all of the files have been copied and the flash drive (baby) is disconnected from the computer (mother), the data contained on the flash drive is the basis for all future use. Though the files can be altered, they are the foundation for everything.

What programs or files are you storing on your internal hard drive? Are there files that you need to delete or alter, new programs to add before you conceive/grow your baby? What messages will you send to your baby? Unintentionally and unconsciously, your mother might have programmed your hard drive with messages that the world was a scary and dangerous place, based on her stress level. Remember, her reaction to her life was based on what she perceived as stressful. Her attitude towards her experiences during pregnancy and the early years of your life formed the foundation of who you are today.

Just as your mother's world-view shaped you, your world-view or attitude will form the foundation for your child's life. For the most part, the subconscious mind is programmed during conception through toddlerhood, which ultimately determines your attitudes and perceptions of your world. This is because the part of the brain that is developed in utero is the thinking and feeling part of the brain. The emotional experiences your child has in the womb direct her brain development as the intellectual part of her brain matures. If your baby has the opportunity to experience the world as a safe and loving place, she can develop a positive mental attitude and her mind will see opportunity. The world is then a place to explore and enjoy. Which will you choose for your child?

Your assumptions are your windows on the world. Scrub them off every once in a while, or the light won't come in."
—Alan Alda

Having a positive mental attitude (PMA) does not come easy or naturally to most people because the subconscious mind is usually programmed for negativity. Why then do you want to put forth the effort? Developing a PMA will not only change your life, but the life of your baby. It changes situations from being annoying, stressful, or even tragic to opportunities for growth. When you focus your energy on seeing the good in life, you will see the good. Looking for the upside of a challenging situation or negative thought can turn "Why are there no parking places near my office?" into "It's a beautiful day for a walk." The world is full of opportunities if you choose to find them. Opportunities are not just for a select, lucky few.

Pregnancy is the perfect time to assess your perceptions and begin to adopt an attitude of gratitude and optimism. Optimistic people attract what they want. They attract good jobs, good friends, and good experiences; the things and circumstances in life that they want. Optimistic people attract positive things and circumstances because they are always on the lookout for them. If you believe that a good life is possible, opportunities will begin to manifest themselves. The Research Project on Gratitude and Thanksgiving, conducted by McCollough and Emmons, found that people practicing gratitude reported higher levels of alertness, enthusiasm, determination, optimism, and energy. They also experienced less depression and stress and were more likely to feel loved. In addition, gratitude releases positive hormones supportive for pregnancy. People practicing optimism actually stimulate different areas in their brain than people who are pessimistic. The optimistic brain is more likely to create a healthy body; optimists are more likely to have healthier immune systems, live longer, are less depressed, and have overall better performance. In fact, studies have shown the hormones related to optimistic thoughts work better than drugs on patients who are clinically depressed. Your brain is a natural pharmacy, which can be used to your advantage for fertility, pregnancy, birth, and breastfeeding. Your body and mind are not separate, nor are your feelings separate from your baby's development.

In fact, optimism can even impact your fertility. One study found that parents who had an attitude of optimism were more likely to become pregnant during in vitro fertilization. Today, many fertility clinics use techniques based in optimism to increase a mother's fertility.

Are you an optimist or a pessimist?

Optimism is defined as a tendency to seek out, remember, and expect pleasurable experiences. Are you seeking happiness? Are you expecting it? If your world-view does not support optimism, it is time to make some conscious change. Why? Consider the child you want to raise, do you want to raise a child who expects happiness and is confident and self-assured, or one who is fearful, anxious, and unhappy? Every mother wants to raise a happy child! You can teach your child to love life, embrace change, and look for the good, even in the unexpected. Research shows us that these teachings begin from the moment of conception. You cannot shelter your baby from your experiences while you are pregnant. Your baby will experience every moment and every thought you have during pregnancy. While you may not be able to change what happens to you, you can change your attitude and reaction to your life. You are in control.

When you become aware of your perceptions, you can change them. You can choose whether to see a storm cloud or a cloud with a silver lining. It may take time and perspective to see the silver lining, but if you believe it is there, it will be. The things you at first perceive as negative can be the catalyst for a great change in your life. Having a PMA is really all about trust. *It is about trusting yourself.* When you trust yourself, you know that in any given situation you have the power to choose how you feel about it. You can choose how or *if* you will react to it. Positive people know that even in the midst of chaos there lies unseen opportunity. When we look for opportunity we find opportunity.

> *Most folks are about as happy as they make up their minds to be.*
> —Abraham Lincoln

People with PMA know that they will be able to have just what they need when they need it. Teaching your child that she can trust that her needs will be met is a wonderful gift you have the ability to give her. From the moment of conception you have the incredible opportunity to be an optimistic, enthusiastic, loving mother.

Baby Steps to Adopting a PMA

The first step to adopting a PMA is recognizing negative thoughts when you have them. This requires active listening to your mind's self-talk. When you catch yourself thinking a negative thought, this is your opportunity to make change. It is not easy to begin to make this shift, nor will you always be aware of your subconscious mind controlling your actions. Every time you recognize a negative thought, this is a gift, an opportunity to become fully conscious. You have an opportunity to experience optimism AND gratitude.

The key to breaking the habit of negative thinking is to use the 3 Rs.

- *Recognize it*: Catch yourself thinking the negative thought. This is actually a moment of mindfulness and awareness. Congratulate yourself.

- *Review it*: Pause and consider the situation. Ask yourself, "Does this situation deserve my reaction or am I reacting inappropriately? Is there another way I can look at this situation?"

- *Replace it*: Take a deep breath, focus on your heart, and consciously think about something else that is positive.

The more that you actively and consciously practice the power of positive thinking, the more it becomes second nature. Help yourself by creating reminders in your daily life to be positive. Place positive quotes on your desk at work, read positive books, seek out positive people who will have a positive influence on you. Pay attention to what and who in your life makes you feel good…as well as what and who doesn't.

If you would like some help developing a positive attitude, there are many great books and techniques available. Here are just a few examples:

- Cognitive Behavior Therapy (CBT): This therapy produces excellent results, particularly in the field of fertility. CBT helps individuals takes situations that may seem overwhelming, and helps break them down into smaller parts so they become manageable. There is evidence that CBT improves attitude and increases fertility; it's a win–win. It has even been shown to return menstruation to women who have ceased menstruating.

- EMDR (Eye Movement Desensitization and Reprocessing): This psychotherapy technique might sound strange, but it has been widely researched and has proven to be a very effective way for people to deal with current or past trauma that may be affecting their lives. It helps to relieve psychological stress, and can be used effectively when there appears to be significant barriers to internal happiness. For more information visit EMDRIA.org.

- Psyche-K: This is a psychological technique used to free the subconscious of mental and emotional barriers that prevent happiness. This technique is based on mind-body medicine, as well as brain research to help undo beliefs that are programmed into the subconscious mind. For more information, please visit www.yourbeliefsmatter.com

Chapter Three
Keys to Mindfulness

"The present moment is filled with joy and happiness. If you are attentive, you will see it."
—**Thich Nhat Hanh**

Whether you call it meditation, prayer, sitting quietly, quieting the mind, or being still, they all achieve the same result: stillness allows you to tune deep within, connect to your source, and become mindful of your internal world. Mindfulness lays the foundation for everything you will learn about having *the greatest pregnancy ever.* You can develop clarity during meditation because you are open to receiving answers to your questions. Meditation is like a two-way radio, as long as you are talking you cannot hear any messages from the other side. You have to stop talking and become quiet to receive messages. Meditation connects you to your subconscious mind, to your source, and allows you to explore your thoughts and beliefs deep within. This exploration also allows you opportunity to deeply connect with your baby.

Meditation, or mindfulness, does not have to mean sitting in a yoga pose and chanting. It simply means having an opportunity to be in a space where you can quiet your mind, move your body into a place of stillness, and connect to your source. Some people find that they can move into meditative states while walking in nature, running, or by simply sitting outside in their garden. There are many ways to become mindful of your internal world.

When you are in a meditative state you release beneficial hormones (neurohormones and neurotransmitters) that your baby will receive through the placenta and later on through breastmilk. These little molecular messengers can help calm your baby, as well as help develop her emotional intelligence by sending her waves of love and other emotions. Meditation also helps the body and mind eliminate stress hormones, which is very important in pregnancy. If you want to do just one thing to benefit the health of your baby during your pregnancy, it should be to reduce stress as much as possible. Meditation is a simple, easily accessible way to eliminate stress, and it is available to you almost anywhere!

Meditation can elevate DHEA, which is known as the mother hormone, because it acts as a precursor to many other important hormones including the male and female sex hormones. It is also an elemental hormone for pregnancy, for without DHEA it's impossible for a baby to grow during pregnancy. It's known as a life-giving hormone. DHEA also increases the effectiveness of the immune system by increasing production of critical immune factors such as t-cells, which are transferred to your baby during pregnancy.

Meditation also stimulates the pineal gland, which secretes melatonin. Melatonin helps you sleep and helps your brain move into alpha states of relaxation. When your brain is in an alpha state your body can easily improve your health through repair, relaxation, and increasing immune function. Additionally, meditation releases endorphins into the bloodstream. Endorphins are naturally produced opiates, which help you feel good and reduce pain. During pregnancy, these endorphins are also sent to your baby.

Meditation lowers the heart rate and blood pressure, which are always beneficial during pregnancy. What could be better than a few moments a day when you send your baby all of the physical benefits of meditation such as immune support, relaxation hormones, and emotional molecules of happiness? It's a gift that will give back to you during pregnancy and after by positively affecting the temperament of your child.

But wait, there's more! Meditation also provides psychological benefits to both mom and baby. Research has associated meditation with creativity, empathy, concentration, and self-actualization. When your mind is calm and you focus your thoughts on love or another positive emotion, your mind begins to release chemical messengers of emotions, called neuropeptides, or molecules of thought. During pregnancy, these thought molecules pulse throughout the body, enter the placenta and then are reproduced and delivered directly to your baby. This is how you communicate directly to your unborn baby. Your baby feels everything you feel. Though your baby is always receiving these thought molecules from you, meditation is a time when you can focus on sending loving, positive, life-fulfilling thoughts to your baby. This is one of the ways emotional intelligence is created in babies. It is how your baby begins to understand emotions and the world. You can positively influence her world by meditating.

Beginners Meditation Guide

Meditation does not need to have many rules. It is simple, though initially will involve conscious effort. With frequent practice, it will begin to become second nature. Sit where you can be warm and comfortable and have at least 5-10 minutes to yourself. You don't have to sit cross-legged or even on the floor, but that is a commonly used meditation position. During pregnancy, as your belly gets larger, it may feel more comfortable to place a folded towel or mat under your bottom. You can also lie down if you need to, just get comfortable.

Once your body is comfortable, allow your spine to lengthen, feel yourself sitting taller. If you lie down, feel your body stretching out. If you wish, rest your hands on your knees or you can place one hand over the heart and one hand over the navel (this is a common pregnancy meditation posture as it helps you connect your heart and your baby).

Once comfortable, just breathe. For a few minutes simply become aware of your breath. Don't try to change it, just notice it. Allow thoughts to enter your mind, but instead of reacting to them just let them go. It is very difficult to have a clear mind when you begin to meditate. Becoming aware of your thoughts and simply observing them (instead of reacting emotionally to them) allows your mind to become calm.

Begin to slow your breath, pausing between each inhale and exhale. Focus your mind on feeling love and gratitude, even if you can only feel grateful for the smallest of things. Stay in this meditative space as long as you can.

More will be shared on specific meditations later in this book, but this is an excellent place to start. The benefits start immediately!

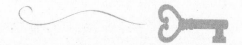

Chapter Four

Keys to Conscious Agreement

"Before embarking on important undertakings, sit quietly, calm your senses and thoughts, and meditate deeply. You will then be guided by the great creative power of Spirit."
—Paramahansa Yogananda

A term you may be exposed to in pregnancy books, your doctor's office, childbirth classes, or the hospital, is "informed consent." Informed consent is a legal term, which means that a patient is consenting to accept a medical procedure, and that she/he has been informed of all the benefits, risks, and alternatives to any treatment offered her/him. This is meant to empower the patient; however, it fails to address the importance of conscious decision-making based on one's intuition, instincts, and gut feelings. Informed consent is made with the mind or intellect. What we ask you to do is to go deeper, past your intellect, into conscious agreement.

What is conscious agreement? It is the act of making decisions based on deep inner listening and coming to an intuitive mind/body/spirit agreement. It is making decisions that feel good at a gut level. Conscious agreement occurs when you are in collaboration with your inner wisdom, when every part of you says, "YES!" It's about moving into a space of trust. This can initially cause anxiety, because when you pay attention and make decisions based on your inner wisdom, you are solely responsible. There is no one else to blame, you are the creator of everything that stems from that decision.

Think of a time when you made an important decision and it did not feel quite right to you. You made a choice even when your inner voice disagreed. Did this decision really work out for you?

Alicia's Story

The women in Alicia's family have all gone to Dr. Washington. He delivered all of the babies in their family, even Alicia. She is now pregnant with her first baby and her mother made an appointment for her to start her prenatal care with Dr. Washington. Alicia talked to the ladies at work and learned about a relatively new birth center that has water birth and natural options available. Her good friend and co-worker Maria just had a baby girl there and has not stopped talking about how wonderful the experience was.

Though Alicia had never even considered having a baby with anyone but Dr. Washington at the regional hospital, she decided to tour the birth center with her husband, Gene. They both thought the birth center felt homey, and they could see themselves welcoming their baby there. When Alicia tells her mother that she is considering the birth center and is canceling the appointment with Dr. Washington, her mother throws her hands in the air and shouts, "Alicia, you're not having this baby with some midwife. How can you even consider having a baby anywhere but at the hospital with Dr. Washington? ALL of the babies in our family are delivered there. Why do you think you're so special?"

Even though Alicia *knows* that having a baby at the birth center feels right, she decides to take the appointment with Dr. Washington. She does not want to cause a family rift; after all, it seems very important to her mother, and she would not want her to have to face Dr. Washington at church. When she tells Gene about her decision, he seems very surprised that she has changed her mind so suddenly. He asks, "Are you sure this is what you want to do?" As she drives to her first appointment with Dr. Washington, she feels like something is off. Her stomach hurts and she has a headache. Is Alicia in conscious agreement?

How do you know when you are *not* acting in conscious agreement?

- When you make a decision and something just feels wrong; when your gut is telling you something is not right. Interesting note: your gut is made up of neural tissue that responds to feelings and emotions. Paying attention to your gut reactions tells you what you think at an intuitive level.
- You continue to question your decision.
- You experience uncomfortable, physical symptoms such as: sleeplessness, stomachache, problems with concentration, a general feeling of dis-ease.

These physical signs are signals designed to alert you that the body, mind, and spirit are not communicating in harmony. Your internal compass is telling you to go in one direction and yet you choose another path. You are functioning in a state of unconsciousness. It is time to redirect.

When you begin to develop the skill of being in conscious agreement for all of the decisions you make, life begins to move towards a different path; a path of less resistance and more opportunity, a place of deep trust and wisdom. Doesn't this sound like a better path to follow?

Steps to Conscious Agreement

Step One: *Separate yourself from external influences.*

This does not mean you have to go on retreat to the mountains. You can do this anywhere, anytime. For example, you can excuse yourself for a breath of fresh air, a bathroom break, or a glass of water and use this time to begin to redirect. You can also simply close your eyes. This separation is important because people often make decisions based on the expectations of others and their subconscious reactions to others. Have you ever noticed that someone else's mood influences your mood? Research shows that your brainwaves actually sync with the people around you. Your brain releases the same hormones as those near you, which cause the both of you to have similar thought patterns. In fact, not only does your brain sync with the brain wave patterns of those around you but so does the beating of your heart. Your heart begins to resonate, or sync itself to those around you, which causes you to experience similar emotions as those around you. The people around you influence you on many levels.

This is called entrainment. Entrainment is often a term used by musicians. Why does the symphony all warm up together? Because when one musician finds the right note, this powerful musical resonance causes the other instruments to begin to synchronize, so everyone is playing in harmony. Our brainwaves and heart rhythms do this as well. When we are around someone sad, we begin to feel sad. Remember the saying misery loves company? The same is true for any emotion, positive or negative. Removing yourself from others when you make a decision ensures that you are making decisions based on your own internal compass, not due to the influence of others.

Alicia allowed the influence of her mother to literally change her mind. Humans have mirror neurons in their brain that cause them to feel the same feelings as those around them. This helps you to "fit in." Unfortunately, it can also cause you to make unwise decisions. Alicia made a decision unconsciously, overriding her gut instincts. Her emotions began to mirror her mother's emotions. Alicia learned long ago and has stored memories in her subconscious that it is better to please her mother and not make waves. She was acting on autopilot and out of habit, instead of staying tuned in to her internal compass.

Between stimulus and response there is a space. In that space is our power to choose our response. In our response lies our growth and our freedom.

—Viktor Frankl

Step Two: *Get quiet and pause.*

Take a moment, or a few, to quiet your mind, breathe deeply, and center your focus on the space around your heart. The Institute of Heart Math has found that when people allow themselves to be tuned into their heart space, they make better decisions.

This step allows you to unplug from all external sources of influence and distraction and plug in to yourself and your own source. Dr. Wayne Dyer, calls this your sacred space. When in your heart space, your only influence is your source, and everything that emanates from this source is good, right, and in your best interest. The heart has a magnetic resonance 5,000 times greater than that of the brain. The heart also has neural tissue, or "thinking" tissue, that causes it to be able to read the environment around you. It has now been discovered that the heart is as powerful as the brain, if not more so, in helping us choose the best course of action based on what is happening around us. Focus in on this heart space before moving to the next step.

Step Three: *Listen in.*

Think of all of the options in front of you. Imagine each one of them. Tune in. How do you feel, both physically and emotionally? Which option feels right? Which option brings you the most peace? (Ask yourself which option brings YOU the most peace, not other people.) It is also important to note that the option that feels right for you may not be the easiest route, in fact it may be a difficult path. Often the difficult paths are those with the best view and they tend to lead to the most personal growth.

Additionally, when pregnant, it is important to honor the motherbaby bond. Your decisions deeply affect your baby and her long-term health and happiness. As you visualize your options, place a hand over your belly and consciously consider your baby. Does this feel right for both of you?

Step Four: *Choose and commit!*

Make the decision that feels right, and commit yourself to that decision. This step is where you begin to make a paradigm shift. You are in control. You make your own decisions. You are responsible. Let go of feeling a sense of guilt for other people's reactions. You are only responsible for your own feelings. Just as you have the opportunity to shift your attitude and choose your emotional response to situations, so do all of the other people in your life. You are not responsible for the feelings of others. At every moment, you have the opportunity to choose conscious agreement for yourself. Having *the greatest pregnancy ever* begins by consciously choosing to live in the moment, and not in the bondage of your subconscious mind.

When you begin to make decisions in conscious agreement you will change the outcome of your pregnancy. Throughout fertility, conception, pregnancy, and parenting you will be faced with daily choices. Making these choices in conscious agreement ensures that you are giving your baby the best that you have to give.

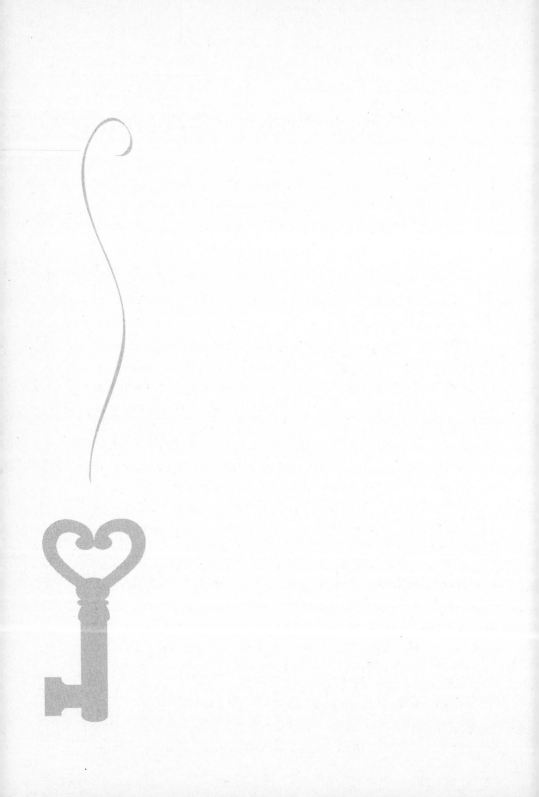

Chapter Five

Keys to Supportive Relationships

"Every issue, belief, attitude or assumption is precisely the issue that stands between you and your relationship to other human beings and between you and yourself."
—Gita Bellin

Relationship to Self

The word relationship brings to mind those people outside of your-self—your partner or another person in your life. However, the most important relationship that you will ever have is the relationship you have with yourself. This is a relationship that begins with self-awareness. You must first love and understand yourself before you can truly love and understand others. There is never a more critical period to love and understand yourself than when you choose to become a parent. Your self-love and relationship to yourself is the very foundation for your child's emotional development. It is true that children learn what they live, and you are your child's first teacher.

How often do you really listen to your thoughts? This is the be-ginning to true self-awareness. Listening to your thoughts with an open mind without judgment allows you to truly become aware of your belief systems. As you grow in self-awareness you will better understand the foundation of many of your beliefs, perceptions, and habits. It allows you to get to know yourself. Examining your thoughts and belief systems gives you an opportunity to look deep inside and think about changing the things that no longer make sense. Knowing yourself, who you are, what you want, and why you want it, gives you an opportunity to move into conscious agreement with yourself and your world. Simply put, no one knows YOU better than YOU. You already have the answers; there is no need to seek external input.

Your beliefs shape every relationship that you have. A deep look at your beliefs, where they came from, and if they are serving you or hurting you is another step towards healthy self-awareness. A belief is when your mind accepts something, whether it is true or not. Your beliefs are generated from the memories of your past. These are the stories you tell yourself to make sense of the world.

> *We build our lives on the foundation of our stories. The more we invest in a story, the more important it becomes to continue investing in that story, even after it is clear the story no longer works.*
> —Bruce Lipton, Spontaneous Evolution: Our Positive Future

What is your story? Are you the conscious author or is your story one that was written a long time ago by other people, events, and things that happened to you? Begin to tell your story as you wish it to be. Create your life with the intentions you desire for you and your baby. Edit your current beliefs if they don't tell the story of the life you want to live and the parent you want to be.

Relationship to Others

Relationships are what the human connection is all about. Your family, your friends and community, your co-workers, your spiritual fellowship, and even your healthcare team all affect how you think, how you feel, and what you do. One of the first critical mothering tasks you have is determining the level of access you will give these individuals to you and your baby. Loving yourself and your baby means surrounding yourself with loving, supportive relationships. This is the time mothers often become conscious of their relationships with others, their relationship with their source, and their relationships with their healthcare providers.

- Who in your life provides you with the support, love, and connection that will ultimately lead to a healthy pregnancy and a happy baby?
- Which relationships in your life should you re-examine?

Who you allow to access your life is very important. You are affected and influenced by the people that surround you. There is no better time than now to start to look at which relationships enrich your life and which relationships keep you from being your best self.

The attitudes of the people around you are contagious. The people that surround you during pregnancy directly affect the health and happiness of the child you will raise. Having conscious relationships is crucial to a happy and fulfilled pregnancy and life. You have the power and responsibility to consciously choose your relationships. It may be impossible to eliminate all unsupportive people in your life, but it is possible to establish firm boundaries.

What are personal boundaries? Personal boundaries are a set of limitations that you have for your physical and emotional health that you expect others to be respectful of. Personal boundaries are healthy and necessary to having *the greatest pregnancy ever*. When you have healthy personal boundaries, you are able to teach your children to have healthy personal boundaries. Creating healthy boundaries means taking an honest look at your relationships. When you don't know who you are and what you want, it is impossible to have healthy boundaries. Does it feel like your relationships are in conscious agreement with who you are, or who you want to be?

Points to Remember:

- It's ok to say "no."
- Tell yourself that YOU and your baby matter most.
- You are not responsible for other people's feelings.
- Others are not responsible for YOUR feelings either, nor should they have to feel the same way about situations that you do.
- Loving someone does not mean you have to engage in a relationship with them.

The Sacred Circle of Support

Imagine yourself surrounded by the people in your life. Take a look around at all of these individuals and select those who are the most supportive and loving in their interactions with you. This is your sacred circle of support, or your inner circle. This inner circle might include your partner, your close family and friends, and those who you consider as your spiritual support team. As you look around your inner circle, notice that these are the individuals who you should keep close to in your life. This inner circle is a sacred space where you are in control. You decide who is in your inner circle. These special individuals are there of your choosing, not just because of their relationship to you or because they are your neighbor or co-worker. They are in this sacred circle because they lift you up and enrich your life. The reason to define this inner circle is to help you identify your boundaries with people in your life. Those in your inner circle should make you feel safe and supported.

Now that you have chosen your inner circle, look at the people in your life who are left. These individuals comprise varying levels of outer circles, based on how close you want to be to them. These outer circles contain people you may wish to have more distance from at times. These people may drain you emotionally, may cause you stress, or you may simply not feel as close to them as those in your inner circle. Additionally, while you may have a deep, emotional connection with some in your outer circle, that connection may not be supportive for you.

Note: Just because someone is not in your inner circle does not mean you don't love them. Your inner circle should simply be made up of those who give positive energy to you instead of taking energy away from you. It is important to recognize whether an individual is in your inner or outer circle when calling on them for support.

Throughout your life your circle of support will change. You change as you grow, therefore your needs change as well as your relationships. Those in your inner circle when you were younger can be completely different from those in your inner circle now. Expect your inner circle to change again significantly when you become a mother. This can be troubling as you begin to realize that your inner circle has changed because you are changing. Out of habit you may call on people for support who should have migrated to your outer circles. Pay attention, and take time to redefine your circles of support as needed.

Gratitude in Relationships

> *We can only be said to be alive in those moments*
> *when our hearts are conscious of our treasures.*
> —Thornton Wilder

When you are in a state of gratitude, your heart is open. It is in this state of gratitude that you are able to give and receive love. The act of gratitude is magnetic. Think of yourself and others as a magnet; you always draw to yourself what you are feeling/expressing. When you are grateful for the relationships you have, others experience that appreciation and love. They are then likely to reciprocate love and appreciation.

Resistance is the opposite of gratitude. It means that you are placing your focus on what you don't want in your life versus what you do want in your life. We get what we give. If you are focusing on behaviors and events that you don't want, you are actually drawing those situations to yourself. Gratitude can be thought of as acceptance. When you are in a state of gratitude (acceptance versus resistance) you are in the optimal state to give and receive love.

Consider these scenarios of acceptance and resistance:

Scenario one: My husband brings me flowers after an especially hard week at work. My reaction is to feel loved and appreciated, offer thanks, and acknowledge his gesture. (Acceptance)

Scenario two: My husband brings me flowers after an especially hard week at work. My reaction is to feel suspicious. Why did he give me this gift? Maybe he has ulterior motives. I ask him "What have you done behind my back that you are trying to compensate for?" (Resistance)

Which of these scenarios opens the door to goodness in your life?

When you are in a state of gratitude, it heightens your perceptions. It opens your eyes to the goodness of life all around you. It changes the way you see people, events, and situations in your world. When you are grateful, you open yourself up to more good, and by opening up to good you attract it. Isn't this the world you wish your baby to be born into, a world of gratitude?

The last segment of this chapter includes activities to help you tap into your subconscious mind and explore your thoughts. There are activities to do by yourself, and also with your partner. These activities are strongly suggested for preconception work or early pregnancy, but can be done at any point in pregnancy.

Part One:

Activities for Be-ing

Belief System

Your family of origin and the memories you hold about your past have a great impact on your thoughts, feelings, and beliefs about yourself. It's important not to underestimate the extent that these beliefs impact your sexuality, fertility, pregnancy, birth, and parenting behaviors. Your core beliefs, like it or not, attract the people, events, and situations in your life. If you have an attitude of fear or shame around pregnancy/birth/parenting this can manifest into fearful and shameful experiences. Many children grow up in families where sexuality and all things related to reproduction (menstruation, pregnancy, etc.) have an element of shame or embarrassment associated with them. This negative perception of your body and the process of womanhood can and does affect the way you conceive, grow, birth, and parent your babies. Often women are unconscious to what they really believe about their bodies and pregnancy because these beliefs are held in the subconscious mind. Here is a list of questions to help you explore your inner-most beliefs so that you can choose to change those beliefs that do not support healthy pregnancy/parenting.

In the exploration of your belief systems and its origins, it is crucial that you recognize the importance of changing the beliefs that do not reflect what you WANT. This exercise is designed to help you:

- Become more conscious of your belief systems and how they were created
- Determine if your beliefs will benefit you and your baby
- Begin to create positive change at a deep level

Recognize that it can be common to move into a state of mind of victimization when you uncover belief systems that don't feel good. Allowing yourself to stay in a state of victimization or self-pity actually wires these beliefs deeper into your subconscious. *It is critical to be committed to change*, and to give yourself an opportunity to move into a state of gratitude or appreciation every time you feel challenged by these beliefs. Notice your feelings (observe them), honor them (do not react to them), and then move into a state of gratitude for what you can. This is being mindful.

It is difficult to do this work. The more you practice changing fears/unwanted beliefs into opportunities, the easier it will become. Uncovering your belief systems presents an opportunity for you and for your baby. When you break the cycle of unwanted beliefs, you change the world and the future for your child and future generations.

Step One: Sit in a quiet space alone and allow yourself to journal freely the answers to these questions. Try not to over-think your answers, or mentally edit them, just allow yourself to write freely as the thoughts come to you. Some of the memories you uncover may be painful or uncomfortable. This is exactly why you want to recognize them and then move into a space of change. After this exercise, if you feel that you need help processing and changing these beliefs, please review the therapies mentioned earlier in Chapter Two. In particular, the technique Psyche-K is specifically designed to change belief systems at a subconscious level relatively quickly.

What things did your family and friends say to you about your body when you were a child? Were adolescence, sexuality, and body changes openly and positively discussed? What feelings do you remember having about your changing body as you grew up?

What did the women in your family share with you or keep from you about their births and their bodies? How did that make you feel?

What did your father or other men/boys in your life say about your body? Pregnancy? Childbirth? Sex? How did that make you feel?

What was the overall attitude towards adolescence, sexuality, pregnancy, and parenting where you grew up? Do you feel it was positive or negative?

Why do you want to have a child? Why do you want to be a parent?

What are your fears about having a child?

What can you give to your child? What do you want to give to your child?

How were babies/children seen in your family? Is this something you want to embrace in your own family? Why or why not?

How do your parents and siblings feel about you having a child? How do your closest friends feel about your pregnancy?

How does your partner feel about having a child? Have you actually discussed his/her feelings or are you assuming these feelings?

Step Two: Now that you have answered these questions, reread your answers. Which of your answers reflect the ideals that you want to pass on to your children? Do your answers reflect who you want to be in this pregnancy and as a mother?

Step Three: Make a list of all the beliefs you wish to change, and why you want to change them.

Step Four: Rewrite the beliefs you wish to change into a positive affirmation.

Affirmations

Affirmations are positive statements of beliefs or truths that reflect your inner intentions. The repetition of writing, as well as saying affirmations out loud, can help to change your subconscious mind when you believe the affirmations have the potential to be true. They affirm beliefs that your inner-most being holds as true, even though at times your subconscious mind may be telling you that they are not. The more you repeat affirmations from a place of gratitude, the deeper they become rooted in your subconscious mind. The key to successful affirmations is practicing them while *feeling* the feeling that you will experience when the affirmations have manifested in your life. Stating affirmations to yourself while in a state of discouragement, irritation, or disbelief will not allow affirmations to change your mind. You must imagine yourself as already experiencing the affirmation and resonate in that sensation for a bit before practicing your affirmations.

Activity One:

Read the following affirmations and select those that seem to speak to you. If you wish, write your own affirmations. Make a commitment to repeat these affirmations to yourself often throughout the day. Write them on your mirror, place them on your fridge, and hang them on your walls. Affirmations should always be stated in the present tense, *I am* versus *I will*. They should be positive and start with the word "I" or "My." Remember to practice them while in a state of gratitude.

Mother:

- My body is strong and capable.
- I am creating a happy, healthy, and loved baby.
- My body is healthy and I am happy.
- I accept that pregnancy and ultimately my labor and birth can unfold safely and as it needs to.
- I am surrounded and connected to love and support.
- I have a loving relationship with my partner and those around me.
- I create my reality and my world is a loving, peaceful world.
- My body is beautiful.
- I experience abundance all around me.
- I am deeply connected to my baby.
- I love my baby.
- I feel gratitude for my pregnancy, my baby, and my family.
- I am safe and secure.
- I can openly and honestly communicate my intimate/sexual needs with my partner.

Partner:

- I feel good about taking care of myself and my partner.
- I have everything I need to provide for and protect my family.
- I see strength in my partner.
- I am grateful for my partner and our relationship.
- I am connected to my baby and my partner.
- I love our baby.

- I offer loving support to my partner freely and often.
- I express love freely.
- I experience abundance all around me.
- I create my reality and my world is peaceful and joyful.
- I can openly and honestly communicate my intimate/ sexual needs with my partner.

Activity Two:

Write out a fear or worry that you have. If necessary, use the previous beliefs activity to identify a fear or unwanted belief. Next rewrite this statement and turn it into an affirmation. For example, change:

"I fear that I will not be a good mother" to "I have all the resources and love I need to protect, nurture and bond with my baby."

Think of something that makes you feel content and grateful. Once you have connected to this feeling, repeat your new affirmation several times a day.

Parenting Intentions

This is the time to begin to understand how you *feel* about issues that will impact you, your partner, and your baby. This section asks you to look at issues related to finances, careers, parenting styles, roles and responsibilities of each parent, religion, cultural traditions, intimacy, implications of extended family relationships, childcare, education, your home, housework, and decision-making. Review these important topics with your partner, so that you can come to a conscious agreement before your baby is born.

How important is our family's nutrition and exercise? How will we support healthy nutrition and exercise as a family?

Who will be primarily responsible for handling the finances of our family? Will you work during late pregnancy? Will you go back to work after the baby is born? Will dad/partner stay at home with the baby? When? How will our family manage any changes in finances? Have we considered unexpected changes in finances?

If you and partner return to work after the baby is born, who will care for the child? Will we have the option of a friend or family member caring for the baby or will we elect to use a daycare center? Have we interviewed or visited any daycare facilities? Are we in agreement on who will be the primary caregiver for our child?

Is your current residence safe and appropriate for a new baby? If not, what are the plans for change? Do your finances support this change? What are all your options for creating a safe, nurturing environment?

What do you want your parenting style to look like? Will you co-sleep with your baby, or will your baby sleep in another room? What does discipline mean to each of you? Will one parent be taking on the majority of the caregiving, or will the responsibilities be divided equally? What are the roles and responsibility of each parent (diapering, feeding, bathing, playing, etc.)?

Have you and your partner decided upon your child's religious/spiritual upbringing? How big a role will religion/spirituality have in your family's life?

Do you and your partner observe the same cultural traditions? If not, have you discussed and agreed upon which traditions will be practiced as a family?

Have you discussed the impact of being a parent on your intimate/sex lives? Will you have a family bed? How will this change your sex life? Do you have a plan to stay intimate with one another?

Which of your extended family will have access to your child? How will you integrate your extended family into your lives? What level of influence do you want your extended family to have on your parenting styles, if any? What boundaries do you both agree will be healthy? Have you considered *your extended family's access to you and the baby during your birth and the postpartum period?*

When will you send your child to school (preschool can start as early as 2 years old)? Will you home school? Will you send your child to private school? Will you have to pay to send your child to kindergarten? Do you plan on starting to save for your child's college education early on?

When your baby arrives, who will be responsible for the housework? What can be left undone? What aspects of housekeeping can you allow friends/ family to help with? Can you hire a housekeeper? Are there any chores that either of you really don't want to do?

What are your plans for the healthcare of your child? Will your family seek out natural healthcare like naturopathy, homeopathy, and chiropractic? Will you seek traditional healthcare? Have you considered things such as immunizations, circumcision, breastfeeding, homebirth or hospital birth, etc? (These topics will be covered in depth in Part Four.)

If you both cannot agree on a parenting decision, who has the final say? What will the process for decision-making look like?

Have you discussed how having a baby will impact your relationships with your friends and your social life? Are there any friends/family members that you think should have limited access to your child? Have you made a plan for that?

Are there any unhealthy/unwanted habits that you or your partner have that need to be changed before the baby comes? What is the plan for change? If change does not occur, what behaviors/habits will not be allowed around the child (drinking, smoking, cursing, television shows, internet access, pornography etc.)?

Part One:
Keynotes for Be-ing

🗝 Be-ing is the act of being conscious and aware of your surroundings and learning how to become a non-judgmental observer in your life.

🗝 Begin to develop and foster a positive mental attitude, PMA. Remember the three Rs to breaking the habit of negative thinking – Recognize It, Review It and Replace It.

🗝 Adopting a mindful approach to life allows you to tune deep within, connect to your source and become mindful of your internal world. Practicing meditation, prayer, and breathing awareness can help you move into a mindful state of Be-ing.

🗝 Conscious agreement is the act of making decisions based on deep inner listening and coming into an intuitive mind/body/spirit agreement. Step One: Separate yourself from external influences. Step Two: Get quiet and pause. Step Three: Listen In. Step Four: Choose and Commit.

🗝 Your relationships are a reflection of your inner world and influence your reality and the health and development of your baby. Developing healthy personal boundaries and practicing gratitude in all of your relationships is a strong foundation for a healthy pregnancy.

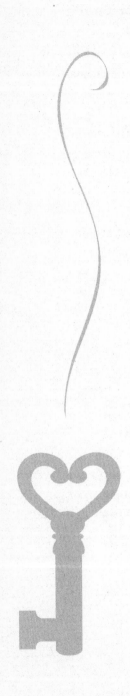

Part Two

The First Trimester of Pregnancy

B-**O**-N-D

O stands for Observing

"Listen to what you know instead of what you fear."
—**Richard Bach**

Chapter Six

What is Observing?

> *"To acquire knowledge, one must study; but to acquire wisdom, one must observe."*
> **—Marilyn Vos Savant**

Pregnancy is a time to begin to become aware of everything in your environment. You begin to pay more attention to what you eat and how often you exercise. You tune in to your relationship with your partner as well as your relationship with your body. How you observe the world will influence your pregnancy and your baby's health. This chapter is not written to make you feel guilty, but instead to empower you with the knowledge that you can make positive change in your life. It is how you *feel* about what is happening in your life that affects your pregnancy and the development of your baby, not what happens to you.

This segment is devoted to *changing your mind*. Changing your mind so that you observe your environment, instead of react to your environment, is one key to a happy, healthy pregnancy. In fact, research shows that a mother's brain is actually changing, creating new connections that allow her to "sense" her environment in new ways. As you begin to become more mindful of your world and create conscious agreement in everything in your life, your baby receives all of the benefits. You will begin to place your focus and your attention on those things that please you, that you are grateful for, and that make you feel fully alive and loved.

Your body is a direct reflection of how you observe the world.

If you constantly perceive your world as a threat, your body reacts with stress hormones and creates *dis-ease*. If you see the world as harmonious, your body is also in a state of harmony. During pregnancy, your world-view is being sent as molecular messages to your baby. This affects your baby's development and your baby's emotional health or EQ (emotional quotient). You have tremendous power and opportunity during your pregnancy to change your life and the life of your baby. When gratitude, peace, and joy are rooted in your state of being, your baby will grow in a state of optimal health.

Your baby becomes who you ARE during pregnancy. Observing all aspects of who you are and who you want to become are the foundational keys to the motherbaby bond during the first trimester. This section of the book includes a look at how you observe the world and how you think about your environment—from stress, to routine medical tests in pregnancy, to common physical discomforts, to the food you eat, to the people and support systems around you.

What's Up, Baby?

Weeks 1–3: Your baby develops into an embryo and implants herself into the endometrial lining of your uterus. The first nerve cells begin to develop. The heart forms long before the brain does. This is due to the fact that the heart is actually the regulatory organ of the body's sensory development. The heart has neural tissue, which helps your baby react and perceive her environment.

Weeks 3–10: The connection between you and your baby, the placenta, has fully formed. Your baby has begun to develop all of her essential organs. Her brain has divided into five vesicles, and 100,000 nerve cells are developing every minute. Her heart starts beating. Her nipples, toes, and external genitals begin to form. Your baby's first sensitivity to touch begins. By the end of this period your baby is moving all around, swallowing, and making hand to mouth movements.

Weeks 10–12: Your baby measures approximately 1–3 inches. Her face and ears have fully formed features. Her limbs lengthen. Her eyelids are formed and closed. She can make a fist. She is sensitive to touch. She responds to your laughter, coughing, and loud sounds. Your baby also begins to determine her sense of balance and her sense of where she is in the world.

What's Up, Mama?

Congratulations! You're going to be a mother! You have missed your period and your breasts may be swollen, sore and tender due to the increase in the pregnancy hormone progesterone. You may have slight cramping or some light bleeding due to the embryo implanting in your uterus. Nausea and sensitivity to smells are common as your body adjusts to the huge shift in pregnancy hormones. In fact, your sense of smell is changing to detect your environment better and your brain is developing new neural connections to make you a more protective and successful mother. Frequent urination is experienced by almost every new mother as your body increases its blood flow and needs to process more fluids. You might feel extremely tired during these first few weeks of pregnancy as your body begins to adjust to the new energy requirements of mothering. Your emotions are often heightened during this time and mood swings are a sign that pregnancy is well on its way, so be gentle with yourself and your loved ones. Towards the end of this trimester you will begin gaining some weight and your pregnancy will start to show. Some women find that they become constipated during pregnancy, especially if they take iron supplements. You may begin craving certain foods, some that you may never have considered before. Your body is seeking nutrition and finds it in the foods you crave. Sometimes mothers crave strange inedible substances like chalk or dirt. These cravings are known as "pica" and can be a sign of a nutrient deficiency, so talk to your care provider if you experience this. It is not uncommon to have vivid dreams during pregnancy, as well as some difficulty sleeping. Your body and mind have become fertile ground. Honor this time by resting, caring for yourself, and your loved ones and nurturing your new relationship to your growing child.

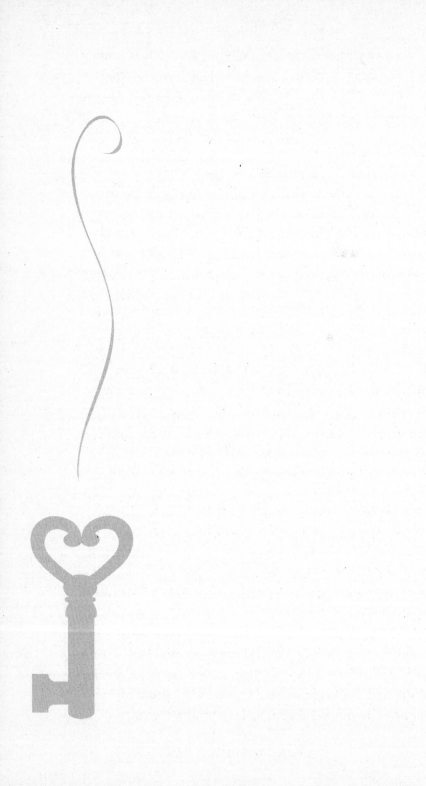

Chapter Seven
Keys to Stress Reduction

"In the end, these things matter most: how well did you love, how fully did you live, how deeply did you learn to let go?"
-Siddhartha Guatama

Stress is simply the body's reaction to unique events in your life. Not all stress is negative. In fact, there is eustress (positive stress) as well as distress (negative stress). Both forms of stress are designed to help the body safely travel through the world. When your body experiences something that demands attention, the body begins to prepare for this new experience. Your brain releases the stress hormones, adrenaline and cortisol, which prepare your body for action. Your body reroutes circulation from its core to your extremities and muscle groups, your heart rate increases, your focus becomes narrow, your blood pressure rises, your digestion slows, and you get a spike of energy. This is often called "fight or flight."

In recent years, for the pregnant woman, this state has been called "tend or befriend" because instead of a mother wanting to engage in a fight or run away, she becomes very task-oriented, increases caretaking activity, and uses her interpersonal skills to negotiate relationships to protect herself and her baby at any cost. These types of activities ensure that mother and baby are in a safe place and well-cared for. This response is the beginning of the mothering instincts. On a personal note, you should avoid staying consistently in a "tend or befriend" state. This means your focus is on taking care of others instead of caring for yourself. Examples include being frequently in a frenzied state of housekeeping, errand running, and chore tending. This is a sign of distress.

Acute or short-term stress, is not harmful for your body, or even your baby in the womb. In fact short bursts of stress, which quickly and completely resolve returning your body to a state of normalcy, actually prepare your baby for stress resiliency throughout her life. What can be damaging to you and your baby's health is when acute stress turns into chronic stress, and your body begins reacting to most things in your environment in a distress mode. During chronic stress, your body continuously releases the stress hormone cortisol, which is not healthy for your pregnancy or your baby. Your body can either make DHEA, the crucial pregnancy hormone, or it can make cortisol, the stress hormone. When your body is busy making cortisol, DHEA production is compromised. Chronic release of cortisol also increases your risk of depression, decreases generation of new cells, reduces memory, and reduces the ability to learn new things (an important skill during parenting).

Perceived stress also impacts the genes of you and your baby. Your genes have telomeres, areas of protection on the end of the DNA strand, which protect the gene's chromosomes from deterioration. When you are exposed to high levels of stress, or chronic stress, these telomeres are damaged. While your baby is developing, ideally she is in a low-stress environment, so that her chromosomes can grow healthy and strong. Interestingly, new research is showing that the enzyme that protects telomeres (telomerase) can be increased by feelings of compassion and acts of care towards others. Pregnancy is a perfect time to offer compassion to yourself, your baby, your family, and your community as your pregnancy hormones, such as oxytocin and estrogen, increase loving feelings. Hugging someone, laughing, deeply listening to someone you care about, cooking and sharing a meal: all these things will benefit you and your baby! It's so simple, really.

Reducing your stress levels can positively impact your pregnancy and your baby. Here are just a few ways lowering your stress can benefit you:

- Healthier sex drive and fertility (important if you are trying to conceive)
- Reduced risk of preterm birth
- Reduced risk of baby born small for gestational age
- Reduced risk of depression in the mother
- Developing a mature hippocampus in your baby (the emotional hub of the brain, which regulates hormones)
- Normal physical development in early infancy
- Increased cognitive scores for your infant
- Normal stress threshold for your baby (babies become stressed less often)
- Reduced risk of your baby's brain becoming habituated, to stress hormones like ACTH and cortisol, which makes her feel unsafe and scared
- Reduced risk of neurodevelopmental disorders (such as autism and schizophrenia)
- Higher IQ
- Decreased behavioral problems in childhood and adolescence

You have the power to improve your life and your baby's life by committing yourself to stress reduction. Rather than becoming more anxious about stress, you can choose to think, "I have the power to reduce the risk of all of these things by taking care of myself. I can quiet my mind. I can take a few moments to do deep breathing. I can take a walk, do yoga, smile, and yawn (a significant stress-reducer). I have all the power. I can CHANGE MY MIND."

The activities just mentioned can change the outcome of your pregnancy. Best of all, they are simple and accessible. Focus on the opportunity you have during pregnancy to make change instead of the risks of being chronically stressed. Things that are proven to reduce stress are: optimism, supportive relationships, meditation, yoga, smiling, yawning, and deep breathing techniques. You also can use the four A's of stress reduction - Avoid, Alter, Adapt and Accept.

Change the Situation

Avoid the stressor – This mean making changes to your environment to keep stress to a minimum. Are you spending a great deal of time with people who cause you stress? Are you participating in activities and events that make you feel stressed out? Learn to say "no" and avoid people and situations that stress you.

Alter the stressor – If you cannot avoid the stressor, how can you change it? Can you modify your hours at work? Can you manage your time better? Do you really need to vacuum the entire house every other day? See how you can team up with co-workers, friends, and family to lighten your load or do these activities with the people you love.

Change Your Reaction

Adapt to the stressor – How can you see the situation in a different way? Are you looking for the good in the situation or staying in a negative frame of mind? Talk about how the situation makes you feel with people you care about, such as your best friend, a counselor, or your spiritual support team. Change how you see things and put the situation in perspective.

Accept the stressor – Sometimes it is impossible to change what is happening or the impact a stressor has on your life. In this case, you can choose your reaction to the stressor even if you cannot change it. Letting go of the need to control the situation can be a big step to reducing stress. When you embrace acceptance, you are no longer in state of resistance and this leads to a more peaceful internal state. An excellent affirmation for acceptance is, "I accept this situation in my life and I trust that all things are working together for my highest good."

Just Breathe

Another excellent way to reduce stress is breathing deeply. Let's hone in on breathing techniques, as they are literally available to you on your next breath. You know how to breathe. Breathing is as much a part of your life as thinking. Learning breathing techniques or "patterned breathing" will not significantly reduce stress. Patterned breath work causes you to use the "thinking" part of your brain. This keeps you from surrendering to your instinctual processes and can actually increase anxiety and inhibit the release of endorphins, your feel-good hormones.

The following exercises were created to help you become aware of *how* you breathe. Most people breathe in shallow, quick breaths as they breathe throughout the day. This is sometimes called backward breathing, and it is an indication of tension and stress in the body. A sign that you are breathing in this manner is that your chest moves more than your abdomen during inhalation and exhalation. The body works best when deep breathing is used, as it stimulates not only the lungs but also the diaphragm, pelvis, abdomen and pineal gland (important for relaxation). This is the type of breathing that will benefit you throughout pregnancy and even in labor. If practiced regularly, deep breathing will become the normal pattern for your breath.

Cleansing Breath

This breath will fully oxygenate you and your baby when you experience a stressful moment. A cleansing breath can also help you move into a state of focus and relaxed attention. It is meant to cleanse the mind and release stress hormones from the body. Inhale deeply through the nose, pause slightly at the top of the breath, and then exhale slowly through the mouth. You can repeat as many times as it feels good.

Belly Breathing or "Deep Breathing"

Place your hands on your chest and inhale as you normally breathe. Notice how your lungs expand. Now place your hands on your diaphragm, just above your abdomen. If you do not notice your hands moving with your breath here, you are using shallow or backward breathing.

Now inhale deeply into your abdomen feeling your belly bulge out under your hands. As you exhale, notice how your hand moves inward toward your spine. Practice this deep breathing, trying to keep your exhale approximately twice as long as your inhale. Some people use a 4/6 count when first practicing deep breathing, inhaling to the count of 4 and exhaling to the count of 6.

As you practice deep breathing, imagine your breath first filling your lungs, then your abdomen, then your pelvis, and the rest of your body, all the way down to your toes. With your exhalation, pay attention to your breath as it leaves the body. Imagine breathing into the space where your baby lies, filling your baby with oxygen, and exhaling any tension that you or your baby may have.

Diaphragmatic Breath with Sigh

Practice the deep breathing techniques mentioned prior, only add a sigh upon exhalation. Inhale deeply through the nose and exhale with a "haaaaa" sound. Sound is a wonderful way to release tension, stress, and even pain from the body.

After practicing this diaphragmatic breath for several minutes, try tightening up all of the muscles in your face, hands, and legs and holding your breath for the count of eight. As you exhale with the "haaaa" sound, allow all the tension you have just built up to be released. Do this several more times. Conclude this exercise by doing deep breathing with your hands on your abdomen, feeling the movement of your breath, and bringing your attention to your baby. This breathwork is particularly helpful to release tension in the body after a stressful encounter.

Three Part Breathing

Practice deep breathing techniques for several minutes. With your next breath, draw your breath first into your belly as much as you can, then into your diaphragm, and finally with the last bit of breath you can inhale deeply into the lungs. Use your hands and feel your belly bulge, then your rib cage, and finally your upper chest. As you exhale, allow your breath to move out of your upper chest first, then your rib cage, and finally your abdomen. This breathing exercise takes some time to master. It is an excellent way to rid yourself of tension and bring awareness into your breathing.

Body Scan with Deep Breathing Technique

The body scan is a technique used to release tension from the muscles in the body and encourage deep relaxation. It is often practiced while lying down. Practice your deep breathing techniques for several minutes. When you feel calm and centered, continue deep breathing and place your focus on your head. Notice any tension around or between your eyes, in your jaw line, or in your tongue. Let go of any tension you feel here. Slowly move your attention down the body. Notice your neck muscles, shoulders, arms, and hands. Soften these areas of the body and feel the tension melting away. Next, bring your awareness to your chest and abdomen, and your low back. Release any tightness in these areas. Then work your way down through your buttocks, thighs, and calves, all the way down through your feet. When you notice tension, bring your awareness to that area and consciously focus on releasing the tension with your breath. This technique, added to deep breathing techniques, can significantly reduce your overall stress. Best of all, these techniques can be done anywhere, even at work.

Smile!

Smiling and yawning are also excellent stress relievers. What could be easier than curling the edges of your lips upwards and bursting into a smile or taking in a deep breath and yawning. It may sound strange but these two behaviors have been found to have profound effects on stress reduction and mood enhancement.

The benefits of smiling include:

- People are kinder and gentler to you
- Calms you down
- Stabilizes your mood, and the mood of those around you
- Creates a feeling of security and happiness
- Feel more sympathetic to those around you
- Smiling is contagious (scientific fact!)

The benefits of yawning include:

- Reduces anxiety
- Increases empathy
- Improves memory retrieval
- Optimizes your metabolism
- Increases your sense of compassion
- Heightens your state of awareness
- Helps you sleep better
- Lowers stress
- Relaxes the body

The Intelligence of Your Heart

Another way to reduce stress is to focus not only on your breath, but the space around your heart (heart space). This allows you to root yourself more deeply in the present and practice mindfulness. The researchers at the Institute of HeartMath have found a variety of stress reducing techniques by simply focusing on the energy of the heart. Many cultures around the world have recognized the importance of the heart for optimal emotional and physical health. Yogic traditions teach about the heart chakra as the seat of balance and consciousness. Religious traditions such as Christianity, Judaism, and Islam also refer to the importance of connecting to the heart for emotional clarity.

Researchers have found that your heart actually "thinks" as it is made up of neural tissue like the brain. It has a separate neurosystem from the brain and does not really even need the brain to function. The heart actually communicates to the brain, and the brain responds. The heart also produces its own hormone, ANF, which is known as the balance hormone. This hormone helps reduce the effects of stress. Even more fascinating is the fact that the heart has an electromagnetic field, which extends out at least eight feet beyond your body and actually communicates with the electromagnetic fields of other people's hearts. Your heart speaks to the hearts of those around you.

This means your heart significantly affects your baby's heart. Heart rhythms tune into one another. This is one reason why you may feel uncomfortable when you are near someone who is in a completely different emotional state than you. That person's heart rhythm feels uncomfortable to you because it is out of sync with your heart rhythm. The longer you are around another person, the more likely it is that your heart rhythms will sync. You literally feel their stress or their happiness. This is another reason why you should carefully select those who are around you and your baby. They can impact you and your baby's emotional state and stress level.

Additionally, your heart rate directly affects the flow of blood and nourishment to your baby via the placenta. A healthy heart pattern and rhythm means a healthy blood flow to your baby. Blood flow to your baby nourishes her, oxygenates her, and removes toxins from her environment.

The heart is the seat of your emotional intelligence, EQ, and is constantly communicating with the emotional centers in your brain. When your heart is out of balance due to negative emotions (anxiety, anger and fear), it creates a disorderly beat and rhythm called incoherence. Positive emotions, such as love, appreciation, and care, create order and harmony in the heart's rhythm, which helps optimize health (*HeartMath Solution*). This is called a coherent heart pattern. These positive emotions are associated with increased immunity, reduced stress hormones, and hormonal balance—all key factors for a healthy pregnancy and a healthy baby.

Your baby's heart develops long before her brain does, and the emotional regions of the brain develop before the intellectual parts of the brain do. Your baby is first an emotional, feeling person, before she is a thinking person. Her feelings make up her world and all that she knows of the world. Pregnancy is the time when you will have the greatest impact on her emotional health.

During pregnancy your baby's brain develops based on your heart and brain wave patterns. The amygdala, the emotional center of your baby's brain, develops according to the state of coherence or incoherence in your body. If your heart and brain are in a state of coherence (experiencing states of love, appreciation, and care), your baby's brain develops to seek out peaceful situations (coherence) for the rest of her life. If your heart and brain are in a state of incoherence (experiencing anxiety, anger, and fear), then your baby's brain develops to seek out chaos to feel "normal." This impacts how your child will navigate the rest of her life—who she develops relationships with and situations she will seek out. Humans always want to feel "at home" and will search out situations, people, and environments that help them feel normal even if that norm is unhealthy. You can help design your baby's brain to look for peace and happiness by cultivating these things in your own life.

To use your heart intelligence to reduce stress, start by becoming mindful of your thoughts, using deep breathing techniques, and focusing your awareness on your heart center. Think about something that makes you happy, someone you love, or something that you appreciate and begin moving into a state of gratitude. The researchers at the Institute of HeartMath have designed specific steps for maximizing your heart's intelligence called Freeze Frame®, Cut-Thru®, and Heart Lock-In®, all very effective techniques. You can find resources through the Institute of HeartMath.

Creativity

Instead of wishing away nine months of pregnancy, I'd have cherished every moment, realizing that the wonderment growing inside me was the only chance in life to assist God in a miracle.

—Erma Bombeck

As mentioned, this trimester is a time to be present and connect to yourself and your baby. A great way for you to do this is by tapping into the creative flow that pregnancy offers. You may find that you feel especially artistic and expressive during your pregnancy. Additionally, taking time to express your creativity can help with stress reduction. One of the reasons you become so creative is because pregnancy and mothering is a right-brained activity. The right hemisphere of the brain is known for regulating empathy, trust, self-awareness, emotion, and stress. It is the creative, holistic part of your brain. The act of mothering is intuitive, spontaneous, and creative, which means that your right brain hemisphere is engaged for better mothering. In fact, your baby will primarily be functioning from her right brain hemisphere in the womb and for the first three years of her life, which puts you and your baby more in tune with one another and promotes attachment. The right side of the brain learns with heart or body knowledge, while the left side of your brain learns from head knowledge. The right side of the brain is associated with feeling and the left side of the brain for thinking. As your right brain hemisphere begins to become more primary during pregnancy and early mothering, you'll find yourself more attracted to artistic activities, more drawn to creative expression.

This discovery is one that can be enormously helpful to you in pregnancy. Tuning in to your inner self can be a powerful way to discover your true feelings, dreams, hopes, and even your fears and worries. Connecting to this part of you can help you through some of these fears and better prepare you for your baby's birth and for being the best mother you can be. You may not feel that you have time to be creative or that it is unimportant compared to your long to-do list. However, allowing time for creative expression helps you become a better mother. So make a date with your baby, put creative playtime on your calendar several times a week during pregnancy.

There are many ways you can express your creativity. You can paint, draw, journal, knit, work with clay, do crafting activities, even cooking can be creative expression. Find something that helps you relax and express yourself. One particularly helpful creative expression for pregnancy is journaling, as it helps you become more connected to your deepest feelings and needs. Gather up some creative tools that you need, such as beautiful paper or a journal and your favorite color pen. This is your artwork and should reflect the inner you, so feel free to use what feels good. Write about your feelings and thoughts often, and spend some time reflecting on what you have written. Keep your journal private so that you can be open and honest with yourself. You instinctively know what you really need and if you journal regularly, these needs will be revealed through your writing. Be gentle and kind to yourself and follow your instincts to connect with your inner wisdom for pregnancy, birth, and parenting.

Remember, it is impossible to live a stress-free life. You can, however, live a life of gratitude and appreciation and learn how to manage the stressful events of life. You choose how you react to the events in your life. These tools will benefit your pregnancy, your baby, your family, and your ability to parent for the rest of your life.

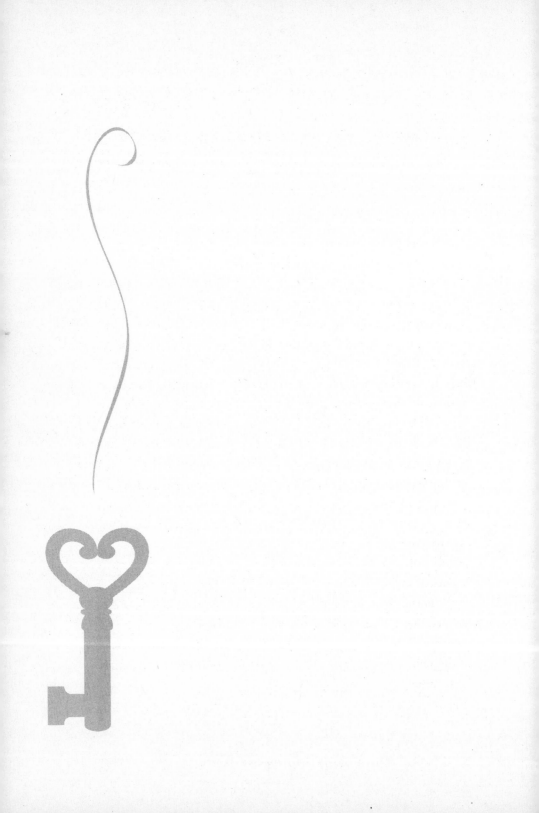

Chapter Eight

Keys to Physical Health for the First Trimester

"Did you ever stop to taste a carrot? Not just eat it, but taste it?
You can't taste the beauty and energy of the earth in a Twinkie."
—**Astrid Alauda**

There is no time like the present to start embracing health in all aspects of your life. Your physical health significantly impacts your fertility, conception, and your pregnancy. Physical health comes from more than just what you eat, drink, and do for exercise. It is impacted by how you feel about your body *and* how you care for it. Making choices that positively benefit your health and your baby's health is a gift that you can give yourself and your family. Making healthy choices in conscious agreement, such as actively choosing a crisp, ripe apple over greasy chips for a snack, allows you to begin to see each moment as an opportunity for vitality, instead of a burden that you are saddled with.

How you feel about the choices you are making is perhaps more important than the choices themselves. The body is an expression of your internal, emotional world. This emotional state directly affects fertility, the health of the developing baby, and the health of your pregnancy. The keys to physical health focus on your observations of the choices you make. The keys are grounded in gratitude and body/mind awareness.

Nutrition

Let's begin with nutrition. This can seem like an overwhelming task, but the reality is the food you eat impacts the health of your body, including the hormones your body releases. Additionally, your nutrition choices change the pH of your body, which can affect fertility, and the health of your pregnancy. The basic rules for eating for fertility and pregnancy are to eat clean, vibrant, colorful foods in as much variety as you can. The following tips can be easily incorporated into your life.

Healthy Weight Gain: Every woman will find that her body needs to gain a different amount of weight during pregnancy, though the average gain is between 25–35 pounds. As long as you focus on eating a variety of healthy, nourishing foods, exercise your body daily, and practice daily breathing activities, your body should be guided to gain the appropriate amount of weight. Surprisingly, your body only needs about an extra 300 calories a day to grow and nourish your baby. Remember conscious agreement when it is time to nourish your body and baby; this technique will help keep you in balance and prevents eating extremes. Pregnancy should not be a time for dieting OR overindulging on a regular basis.

The following is a guide to show you the average weight gain of different body parts during pregnancy:

BODY PART	POUNDS
Blood Volume	*3 Pounds*
Breast Tissue	*2 Pounds*
Uterus	*2 Pounds*
Baby	*6.5-9 pounds*
Placenta	*1.5 pounds*
Amniotic Fluid	*2 Pounds*
Fat and Protein	*7 Pounds*
Water	*4 Pounds*

Eat Clean and Natural: Eating foods that are organic, natural, and not processed allows your body to make maximal use of the properties in the foods. The typical mass-produced vegetable contains chemicals, waxes, and pesticides that can affect your fertility, your developing baby, and even your milk when you are breastfeeding. When choosing meat and dairy products, which can be important sources of protein for pregnancy, try to choose pasture-raised animals that have not been exposed to growth hormones. Cage-free poultry and eggs have higher amounts of omega fatty acids, which is critical to the implanting embryo and developing baby. Omega fatty acids are called essential fatty acids because they are essential to healthy development. Choose fish that are less likely to be laden with mercury such as: sardines, anchovies, wild salmon, and flounder. Eating fish rich in omega fatty acids will also help you think better! Fish to avoid or eat in very limited quantity include any farm raised fish (such as tilapia), shark, swordfish, king mackerel, and yes, tuna. It may sound strange, but eating fresh foods that will rot quickly is better for you, because it means they are not filled with preservatives and trans fats. Most packaged and fast foods are loaded with preservatives and unlikely to rot any time soon. Foods with trans fats should be avoided as often as possible.

Enjoy Healthy Oils: Yes, it's true, many oils and fats are good for you, especially during pregnancy and for fertility. The latest USDA food guide, called MyPlate, encourages pregnant women to include healthy oils in their diets. In fact, oils high in omega fatty acids enhance ovulation. Though oils should be eaten in consciousness, they are still part of a healthy pregnancy diet. Avoid most oils on the grocery store shelves because they have been processed and are often rancid. The best oils for cooking are coconut oil, ghee (clarified butter), organic butter, peanut oil, and high oleic sunflower and safflower oil. Oils such as olive oil, grapeseed oil, flaxseed oil, and walnut oil are best for tossing on salads and drizzling over veggies. These oils change their chemical makeup when exposed to heat and light and lose their health benefits.

Even better than drizzling foods with healthy oils is to eat the natural source—eat a nut, crack open a coconut, snack on seeds, eat an olive! Additional important sources of healthy fats are avocados, flax seeds, and clean, small fish or bottom-dwelling fish (anchovies, flounder, sardines, and salmon). Most oils should be kept only a couple of months and should be stored in dark bottles in a cool place. Only buy what you need! Buy organic, as most pesticides are fat-soluble, which means pesticides can accumulate in high quantities in pressed oils. One of the best things you can do to improve your health is to throw away any and all margarine in your refrigerator. If you need buttery flavor, use real butter or use ghee (found in most health food stores), just use small amounts. The hydrogenated oils (trans fats) in margarine are bad for your growing baby's brain and neural system development. Your baby's brain will be sixty percent fat by weight, so supply her with healthy brain-building fats!

Nosh On Veggies! Most vegetables are alkaline foods, and this supports a healthy environment for conception. An acidic environment is not friendly to sperm. If you are trying to get pregnant or are in the early weeks of pregnancy, focus on alkaline-rich foods, not acidic foods (like meats and dairy). Examples of alkaline foods include dark, leafy vegetables, almonds, asparagus, and mangoes. You can find many alkaline food charts on the internet. Munch on cruciferous vegetables, such as broccoli, cauliflower, Brussels sprouts, radish, bok choy, kale, collard greens and watercress, which contain di-indolylmethane. This helps the body metabolize estradiol, which allows for more effective use of estrogen, necessary during fertility, conception, and pregnancy. Eat veggies with deep, rich colors, because they have more micronutrients and phytochemicals, which will help protect your ovaries and your baby from free radicals, which damage cells. Vegetables are important throughout pregnancy. The darker, more colorful varieties are more flavorful and loaded with nutrients.

Don't Forget Your Vitamins and Minerals! These are especially important to fertility and pregnancy. If you manage to eat a varied and nutritionally balanced diet, there is no need to supplement. However, most mothers have days they want to order french fries, forget to pack a plum in their lunch sack, or choose to snack on chips instead of broccoli, so complementing your diet with a multivitamin supplement is a good idea for most. Vitamins A, C, E, B complex (including folic acid), zinc, and selenium are important to fertility and pregnancy, so find a whole food vitamin that contains these nutrients. Folic acid is particularly important during the first trimester, when your baby's neural system is developing.

Whole food vitamins, as opposed to synthetic vitamins (most over-the-counter vitamins), are produced from real food, not created from chemicals in a lab. Your body knows how to process whole food vitamins and get the most out of the nutrients they contain. Whole food vitamins contain vitamins and minerals in a natural food state, meaning they are found with companion nutrients that help your body digest them better. They are also less likely to cause nausea and stomach upset. Synthetic vitamins can contain toxins that can accumulate in your body and your baby's body. Go natural! Many doctors unknowingly offer prescriptions for prenatal synthetic vitamins because they are unaware of the potential side effects and physical discomforts they cause, such as constipation and increased nausea. Check with your care provider about which whole food vitamin alternatives they might suggest (or talk to a nutritionist or natural healthcare provider who specializes in pregnancy).

Some women find their bodies need more iron as their blood volume increases. Natural iron supplements like Floradix can be easier on the pregnant body than synthetic iron supplements, which can cause constipation. Excellent sources for vitamins and minerals are juicy fruits and vegetables. Snack on apples, mangoes, raspberries, and blueberries. Typically, the deeper the color of a fruit or vegetable, the more nutrients and antioxidants it contains. Flash-frozen fruits are a great substitute when fresh fruits are not readily available. Try a greek yogurt and berry smoothie for a mid-morning snack instead of relying on a candy bar for energy. It will deliver great nutrition and satisfy your sweet tooth!

Avoid No-value Foods: No value foods include sugar, white flour, and white rice, which turn quickly into simple carbohydrates that do nothing to enhance your health. If you must sweeten your food, avoid ALL chemical sweeteners such as aspartame, saccharine, and sucralose. Long-term studies have not shown these chemical additives to be safe for pregnancy, so it's best to avoid them. Better options are maple sugar, honey, and natural stevia (not chemically-enhanced stevia products). White sugar also elevates stress hormones, something you want to avoid in pregnancy.

When you begin to replace white flour products with whole grain alternatives you will begin to see how delicious real grains are. Better alternatives for no value grains are barley, oatmeal, buckwheat, quinoa, amaranth, brown rice, and wild rice. These are all delicious alternatives to white starches, and they are filled with vitamins. Make a double or triple batch of healthy grains when you cook them so you can store the extra and have some on hand for easy sides and salad mixes throughout the week.

Tip: Shop the perimeter of the grocery store, as well as the tops and bottoms of the store racks (instead of the middle, eye-level rack) where healthier, non-processed foods tend to be. Grocery stores tend to place their high cost, super processed foods near the entry and in the center the store, knowing that it will entice you to purchase these items.

Move Your Body! Exercise and movement are part of a healthy pregnancy. The simple act of movement sends nourishing blood flow throughout your body, to all of your organs, and to your growing baby. Movement also helps remove stress hormones from your body. It lubricates your joints. Movement makes you feel good, and as pregnancy progresses it can alleviate many aches and pains. Exercise is also a natural antidepressant. Commit to some sort of body movement at least thirty minutes a day. Whether it is a walk, yoga, a hike, dancing, swimming, or a prenatal exercise class, just move!

Prenatal yoga is a wonderful way to bring your body, mind, and spirit into a deep state of connection. Yoga allows you to practice mindfulness and begin to cultivate a non-judgmental, accepting attitude about your body and your life. As your body grows with pregnancy, yoga helps you develop a love and acceptance of your changing body. The practice of prenatal yoga has been shown to increase mobility; improve circulation; reduce certain pregnancy discomforts such as backache, heartburn, and sciatica; reduce blood pressure; elevate your mood; and improve sleep. Prenatal yoga has also been associated with reduced stress, reduced preterm delivery, healthy birth weights, and fewer birth complications.

The general goals of prenatal yoga are:

Enhance body awareness as changes of pregnancy occur

Help alleviate certain physical discomforts, such as backache

Evoke deep relaxation states

Develop flexibility, strength, balance, and agility

Nurture community

Learn to cope to with stress in healthy ways

Develop comfort measures to cope with labor and birth

There are certain complications in later stages of pregnancy that are considered contraindications for the practice of prenatal yoga. In the event that you experience any of these symptoms, you will want to talk to your healthcare provider before continuing your yoga practice. They include ruptured membranes, persistent bleeding, placenta previa, pre-eclampsia or toxemia, early cervical dilation, and uncontrolled cardiovascular disease. Most mothers in relatively any stage of fitness can participate in a prenatal yoga class and find many benefits. Always check with your healthcare provider before initiating any new form of exercise.

Prenatal yoga can help you as an expectant mother connect your body, mind and spirit. This ancient practice allows you to tune in to your body as it begins to transform. Yoga invites you into a world of balance, peace, and mindfulness. If possible, try and find a class where you can meet other moms and have an experienced teacher help usher you through your pregnancy.

First Trimester Physical Changes

Please check with your healthcare provider about the safety and efficacy of any treatment for physical challenges in pregnancy.

Morning Sickness: Morning sickness, or prenatal nausea, is often your body's reaction to the increasing hormones being produced during pregnancy. Unlike its name, it doesn't only happen in the morning and can sometimes extend throughout the entire pregnancy. Morning sickness is normal, and it means that your body is producing healthy pregnancy hormones. Ways you can cope with morning sickness effectively and holistically include:

- Drink peppermint or spearmint mint tea, or use Grade A essential oil of peppermint for aromatic use.
- Drink homemade ginger tea, natural ginger ale, or eat real ginger candy.
- Use acupressure. You can wear specialized wristbands, often used for seasickness, which stimulate the pressure point P6 (pericardium 6) located on the inside of the wrist. Pressure on this area is known for relieving nausea. Additionally, there are several other good anti-nausea points on the body. Check with an acupuncturist for the best pressure points for your situation.
- Take a vitamin B supplement in the morning and at night.
- Care for yourself by receiving chiropractic treatment, mas-

sage, and reflexology.

- Smell a lemon, or keep Grade A essential oil of lemon around for aromatic use.
- Take two teaspoons of apple cider vinegar in warm water in the morning.

In extreme case of morning sickness, referred to as hyperemesis gravidarum, some women may need prescription medication and/or IV support. Check with your healthcare provider if morning sickness goes unresolved, or if you are experiencing weight loss as a result of nausea.

Fatigue and Insomnia: Your body is undergoing immense physical and hormonal changes at this time. It is normal to feel tired, and yet you might also find it difficult to sleep. This is a time to slow down. Look at your schedule and see what you can eliminate. It is common for mothers to want to do, do, do and go, go, go during pregnancy to get things done so they feel ready for the baby. However, always being on the go is linked to increased stress, insomnia, and exhaustion. Things you can do to help with fatigue and exhaustion are:

- A daily practice of meditation and deep breathing techniques
- Hypnosis for pregnancy
- Practice the Alexander Technique (Find a trained practitioner to teach you.)
- Receive regular prenatal massage
- Prenatal yoga
- Aromatherapy with lavender, roman chamomile, orange, and rosemary verbenon
- Bach Flower Remedy® or Rescue Remedy®
- Sleep with an herbal pillow that contains any combination of lavender, chamomile, lime flowers, and hops
- Have a warm cup of raspberry leaf tea

Frequent Urination: The need to go to the bathroom even when your bladder may be relatively empty is the result of pregnancy hormone hCG, human chorionic gonadotrophin. The pregnant body is cued to filter more wastes and process more fluids. This causes your kidneys to work harder. This uncomfortable side effect of pregnancy may be a challenge, but try to be accepting of your body's unique ability to support the life of another person inside of you. Don't skip bathroom breaks, listen to your body, and go to the bathroom when you have the urge. Cystitis, or urinary tract infection, is more likely to occur if you hold off urinating when you need to go. This is simply one of the ways the body begins to teach us to tune in to our needs, and in the future, the needs of your baby. You can help eliminate the risk of stress incontinence (when urine leaks out when you cough, laugh, sneeze, or exercise) by practicing perineal floor exercises, sometimes called Kegel exercises. In yoga, this practice is called engaging the mula bandha (pronounced: moo-la bah-nd ha).

What you can do:

- Avoid diuretic drinks and caffeinated beverages like sodas, dark teas, and coffee.
- Practice engaging your mula bandha. This is called the root lock. It is said to ground and root the body and allow your energy to flow into the central channel of the body. Engage the muscles between the anus and the genitals (the pubococcygeal muscles, or pc muscles) and lift those muscles upwards towards the spine. This action strengthens these muscles, which act like a basket of support for the reproductive organs, the bladder, and the kidneys. Strengthening these muscles will help tone your internal body, and later, help with the birth process and postpartum healing. Practice engaging these muscles and holding them to a count of ten several times a day. To do this, close your eyes and tighten the muscles around your

anus and hold. Then bring your attention to the muscles inside the vagina (these are also the muscles you use to stop the flow of urine), tighten them, and lift them. Hold tightly all of these muscles, from the rear perineal floor muscles to the front, and feel these muscles lifting upwards. You can also practice fluttering the pc muscles by flexing rapidly, or engaging and releasing in quick succession.

- Stay hydrated, but avoiding drinking large amounts of fluid right before bedtime.
- Urinate when your body tells you to.
- Wear a sanitary pad if you experience urine leakage. Be sure to check with your healthcare provider to ensure it is not amniotic fluid or a vaginal infection.
- Call your doctor or midwife if you experience pain or burning during urination, have a fever, see blood in your urine, or feel the need to urinate immediately after going to the bathroom.

Skin Changes: Your hormones are changing, and therefore every part of your body responds to these changes, even your skin. Here are some common skin changes:

- Acne: You may experience an increase in facial oils and either develop acne or see it resolve. Take care of your skin. Remember that your skin is your body's largest organ. Everything you put on your skin gets absorbed into your body. Consider using certified organic products on your skin. This can be more challenging than it seems because nearly three quarters of all skincare products on the market contain chemicals that are dangerous to your growing baby and you, including the ones you may receive at the hospital. Read the labels! Most skin care products contain carcinogens (cancer causing agents), teratogens and mutagens (which cause birth and cellular defects), reproductive toxins (increase risk of male and female infertility), developmental toxins (harmful to fetal development), skin toxicants, and allergens. Ingredients specifically to avoid include: mineral oil, petroleum products, propylene glycol, and lauryl sulfate. Please note that Accutane, a medication for acne is NOT SAFE for pregnant women. If you have a prescription for this drug, talk immediately to your healthcare provider.

- Chloasma: The mask of pregnancy. Some women experience a darkening of the pigment of their skin on their face. It is more common in women who have pale skin and dark hair. Avoid long exposure to sunlight and use safe, PABA-free sunscreen. The mask usually goes away completely after pregnancy.
- Linea Nigra: This is a darkening line of pigment from the navel to the pubic area. It fades and goes away after pregnancy.
- Spider veins: Due to increased blood flow and circulation all around the body, as well as hormonal changes, some women get spider veins. These tiny blood vessels may look like red patches on the skin. They usually go away after pregnancy.

Sinus Congestion and Nose Bleeds: As your circulation increases and hormones flow through your body, the nasal passages and membranes may become swollen and cause uncomfortable congestion and nose bleeds. Here are some ways to alleviate discomfort:

- Use a neti pot twice daily to moisten your nasal passages. The neti pot is filled with warm, purified salt water. The end of the vessel is placed in one nostril and then water is slowly poured from one sinus cavity out the other. It may sound strange, but it is a very gentle way to cleanse and moisten your nasal passages.

- Avoid blowing your nose often. Instead, use a neti pot to cleanse your sinus passages.
- Use saline drops for moisture in your nasal passages.
- Place warm, moist washcloth or compress over your nose and cheeks.
- Use a drop of Grade A essential oil of lavender, helichrysum, or geranium on your nose and the base of your neck.
- For nosebleeds, place a drop of one of the essential oils mentioned previously on a tissue, wrap around an ice chip, and place under your upper lip, pressing in towards your nose. Alternatively, use an ice pack on the bridge of your nose to reduce swelling. Avoid pinching your nose, as it can cause bleeding down the trachea.
- Use acupressure for sinus pressure. Place your thumbs on the outside of the bridge of your nose pressing into the underside corner of your brow. Lean forward and rest your elbows on a table so your thumbs put pressure on these points. Rest here for a few minutes and practice deep breathing.

Your body is communicating with you throughout your pregnancy. Take time to listen in and pay attention to your body's needs. Ultimately it will lead to a healthier pregnancy and a happier you.

Chapter Nine
Keys to Support in Pregnancy

"Call it a clan, call it a network, call it a tribe, call it a family.
Whatever you call it, whoever you are, you need one."
—Jane Howard

Your family, your friends, your co-workers, your spiritual support team, and your healthcare team will all be part of your support system. Even as early as the first trimester, your relationships will impact your developing baby because your relationships impact your belief systems and your stress level. Now is the time to focus on your most supportive relationships and observe your relationships with friends and family, your community, your healthcare providers, and your source/higher power. Who in your life provides you with the support, love, and connection that will ultimately lead to a healthy pregnancy and a happy baby?

Your Family

If you think you are so enlightened, go spend a week with your parents.
—Ram Dass

Even though you do not get to choose your family, you do get to choose the relationship that you have with your family. This becomes even more important when you are expecting a baby because these relationships will not only affect your life, but will affect the health of your growing baby. When observing your relationships with your extended family, it is common to believe that there is nothing that you can do about those relationships that feel unsupportive. You may think that you must tolerate these unsupportive relationships or that you have no control over them because they are with family members. Remember that you are always in control of who you allow to be part of your life. It may also be true that you have wonderful relationships with your family members, but still need to create some boundaries.

Pregnancy is an opportunity to observe the impact that your important relationships have on your life. You can consciously choose to create a deeper bond with those who positively impact you, or you can choose to limit your relationship with those that have a negative impact on you, depending on how you feel when you are with them. Familial relationships begin when you are growing inside your own mother, and continue to form in the early years of your life. These relationships become embedded in your subconscious. It is important to be aware of this as you are growing and nurturing your child during your pregnancy. How do you want your child to begin her relationships with these people? It all starts with how you see your extended family now, and how you *feel* about each person. Your perceptions of your family become your child's perceptions. The current health of your relationships with your extended family is the basis for the health of the family you are creating. Take some time in the next few days to really consider this.

Are your relationships generally gratifying, loving, and nurturing? If so, you should focus on spending more time and energy on these relationships. Are your relationships a source of anger, anxiety and stress? Is it time to start healing and open yourself up to forgiveness? Do you need to limit contact with these individuals? In emotionally/ physically abusive situations, you may need to completely end your exposure to certain family members, and create healthy/safe boundaries for you and your baby.

Regardless of any boundaries you decide to create, there are often lingering emotions and past experiences that can be healed by forgiveness. Forgiveness is about freeing yourself from the bondage of negative emotions you feel towards someone; forgiveness is not about absolution of guilt. Choosing to forgive does not change the past; rather, it frees you from the negative emotions of past events. It puts the power back in your court; no longer will the person or event hold power over you. A little forgiveness can go a long way and it can help you to forge a healthier connection with the individual in question. Wouldn't you prefer for your child to have deep, loving, healthy, and happy connections in her life?

> *To forgive is to set a prisoner free and discover that the prisoner was you.*
> -Lewis B. Smedes

For those family members (and, really, anyone in your life) that cause you to feel stress and anxiety, it is important to *change your mind* in order to change the way you feel about that person. It is not enough to simply acknowledge a negative emotion that you feel about someone close to you. These emotions still are connected to your baby. You must begin to see the relationship in a new light.

Try this exercise:
Sit for a moment, close your eyes, begin your deep breathing, and bring a vision of the person who you feel negative emotion for into your awareness. Acknowledge the feeling you harbor for them. Notice how those emotions feel in your body. Notice how your body reacts. Does it feel good? If not, make note that your baby also feels these uncomfortable sensations. Your baby is first a feeling human and only later becomes a thinking human, so every emotion you feel becomes your child's world. Are you ready to change these negative emotions?

Take a deep breath. Envision that same person, and this time see them surrounded with light. Offer unrestricted love to them. Pick out something that you feel grateful for in this relationship or as a result of this relationship, no matter how small. Focus on that feeling of gratitude. If it is impossible to feel gratitude, ask for help from your source. Ask, "Please help me see this person, this situation, in a more loving, peaceful way." Wait a few moments. If you still feel anxiety, just focus on your heart center, breathe, and stay in the space of gratitude you have created for this person. Practice this technique every day and you will begin to see your relationship to this person change. It is not your family that causes you anxiety. It is how you *SEE* your family that causes your reaction. The boundaries that you create around your family and how you *react* to them are what cause the anxiety and stress that you experience.

Key concepts to remember when dealing with your family during pregnancy:

- You are influenced by your subconscious programming. More often than not, your actions are guided by your past experiences. Few people are aware of this. You can always choose compassion and love as a basis for any action you take. Always ask yourself, how can I see this person/situation differently?

- Your relationships with your family will change when you stop reacting to your own subconscious programming. Stop, look, and listen. How do you feel about this person when you place them in your heart space? Does it change things for you?

- You have no control over other people's actions. You cannot change your family. Wishing things will change is wasted energy. You can only change your response to them and how you see the situation.

- Let go of the desire to have your relationship with your family look a certain way. Instead, accept the way things are and find ways to be grateful for what those relationships bring to you and your growing baby.

Chapter 9

Your Friends and Community

Humans need each other. Research shows that people who are part of a social network live longer and are more likely to survive life-threatening diseases. People who have a close circle of friends are more secure and have a greater sense of well-being. It's easier to navigate through life's many choices when you know you are being supported.

Becoming a parent will change your friendships. Some friendships will deepen as you move into parenthood and become even more valuable and meaningful to you than they are today. Other friend-ships will all but fade away. This is a very normal part of becoming a parent. Pregnancy and early parenthood will present opportunities to make new friendships and bonds that support your new lifestyle as a parent and as a family. Before you know it, your child will be a catalyst for making new friends too. You will meet families at the park, at your child's school, and even at the local play area. Many new families find that having friends with children around the same age makes life much easier. When there is trust and support between friends, it creates opportunities to help each other with childcare, share resources, provide emotional support, etc. Particularly during pregnancy, it can be helpful to connect with women who are going through the same physical and emotional changes.

This does not mean that you have to give up your friends who do not have children, your single friends, or even your fun-loving, crazy friends. It does mean that your life is going to change. When you find that a friendship seems to be moving further out of your daily life, it is important to focus on the value and the feelings that the friendship once brought to your life instead of the sadness or disappointment of this loss. Life is constant change. Many new parents find that after they have children certain friends take more of a backseat role in their lives, and communication becomes less frequent. This loss of contact should not be taken personally. Some people are just not comfortable with babies and children, but that is not a reflection on how they feel about you or your child. Spend some time feeling appreciation and gratitude for what that relationship brought to you. Remember to value each day for what it is, live in the present, and look for opportunities for new friendships as well as strengthening the friendships that are supportive to you at this time in your life.

Connecting with other expectant mothers during pregnancy is a wonderful way to fully come into motherhood. There are a variety of classes designed for expectant women such as pregnancy exercise classes, prenatal yoga classes, childbirth classes, breastfeeding classes, and other types of support groups. By attending classes while you are pregnant, you give yourself the chance to meet other people who can relate to what you are going through. Resources and information can be shared, and life-long friendships can be made. Mothers also enjoy cyber relationships through online forums, where women can engage in discussions and share resources.

Your Co-workers

Many pregnant women spend a significant amount of time with co-workers, at least a few days a week. On an intellectual level, it may seem as though you have no control over who your co-workers are and how you have to interact with them. It is important to realize that, like it or not, co-workers influence your daily life. Being aware of this fact is important to the health of your pregnancy because your interactions with co-workers can either help contribute to your healthy pregnancy or add to your stress level. You may spend forty-plus hours a week with co-workers and therefore, they will have a significant impact on your pregnancy.

There may be a co-worker in your life who gossips, complains, and emanates negativity. While you cannot control these people or avoid them completely, you can control how you let them affect you. You can choose not to emotionally engage with anyone who isn't supportive of a peaceful lifestyle and pregnancy. Try to become aware of any co-worker who creates drama or negative energy. Once you are consciously aware of who these people are and how you are affected by their behavior, you can take steps to change your mind about how you see this person and/or minimize any contact with them.

Changing your mind about how you feel about someone is not really as hard as you think. The first step is to begin to see how you are a participant in the actions that make you feel unhappy/stressed. Do you choose to participate in gossip? Do you choose to take things your co-workers say personally? Do you let things like reports and deadlines weigh down your heart, instead of allowing yourself to focus on what is really important in your life? Have you tried seeing your co-workers through your "heart space?"

Have you placed the priorities of your life in the right order? For many people, once you really look at your life, priorities will often (though not always) break down something like this:

- Your relationship to yourself, your spirit, and/or your connection to your source
- Your relationship to your baby
- Your relationship to your family and partner
- Your relationship to your friends
- Your relationship to those things that nourish you and sustain your soul
- Finally, your job and your relationships with co-workers

When your priorities are out of order, it is easy to let your relationships with your co-workers have an artificially inflated importance.

Your next option is to minimize contact with co-workers who cause you to feel stressed. When negative situations with these individuals occur, remember that you have the power to choose how you react. You can observe their behavior in consciousness and choose not to plug-in. Talking with, or reacting to, these people only multiplies the negativity. When conversation starts to descend from real work-related information into gossip or blame, remove yourself. Take a quick five-minute break, breathe deeply, and envision your baby's beautiful face. Focus on your heart space. Once the negative co-worker realizes that you won't plug in, they are less likely to try and engage you into their future drama. Dr. Wayne Dyer often says, "When you change the way you look at things, the things you look at change." Begin a work atmosphere renovation. You might even place a sign near your desk that says, "Baby construction zone—no negativity!"

Everything and everyone around you affects your baby's development and the person she will become. By choosing to spend time with your positive co-workers and/or choosing to view your negative co-workers in a different light, you are choosing to have a less stressful workplace and a healthier pregnancy for you and your baby.

Your Spiritual Support

Pregnancy is a time when you begin to make observations about who you are, why you are here, and how you want to raise your children. It's a time you may seek out or deepen your spiritual connection and spiritual support. Spiritual support means something different to everyone. Simply put, your spiritual support can be anyone or anything that helps you feel connected to your source, that which gives you purpose. Your support can be a traditional church and clergy, or it can be an activity that is very private and just between you and your source. Whatever means of spiritual support you seek, it should provide you with comfort and peace, not become a source of guilt and shame. You may want church attendance to be a tradition/ritual that you instill in your child. Being a part of a congregation of like-minded people may offer you support and comfort. However, you may find a private relationship with your source feels more spiritual and connective to you. For example, some people use various forms of meditation, such as silent prayer, mindful breathing, or ritual, as their connection to their source.

No matter how you choose to connect to your source, what is vital to your pregnancy and the development of your baby is that you do find a deep connection to your source. You want to find and connect to whatever it is that provides you with joy, love and connection. There are really only two ways of functioning in the world: acting in fear or acting out of love. Deepening the connection to your source during pregnancy helps you to act from a loving space. When you are acting out of love, you are at peace and the womb is also a peaceful place. This is the best environment for your baby.

Ask and it shall be given to you, seek and ye shall find, knock and it shall be opened to you.
-Matthew 7:7, The Holy Bible: King James Version

Science has recognized the real power of prayer and meditation in positively influencing the body and mind. There are benefits no matter what theological belief system the prayer stems from. Taking moments to become quiet and connect to your source offers amazing benefits. The keys to successful prayer and meditation according to recent research are as follows:

- You must believe in your connection to source when you pray or meditate
- Prayer is not about asking for something from your source, rather, it is about surrendering the situation to your source to allow the highest good to manifest
- Prayer connects you to the loving influence of your source
- Non-directed prayer (praying for whatever is in the highest good of all versus a direct prayer, which is asking for something specific) has the most potential for change and love
- Prayer is limitless, timeless, and always available

...May your Spirit, which is within me, so guide my thoughts, my feelings and my perceptions of all things that I might grow into a happier, more peaceful, more loving human being. Illumine my mind, illumine my life. Amen.

-Marianne Williamson, Illuminata: A Return to Prayer

Your Healthcare Team

You will be surrounded by healthcare providers who will care for you during your pregnancy, as well as after your baby is born. Conscious agreement and a personal connection with these individuals will help you feel loved, cared for, and supported, which has an impact on the health of your pregnancy and baby. Often women select pregnancy care providers based on insurance limitations, convenience of location, or past/current healthcare providers with whom they already have a relationship. The average expectant mother spends less than fifteen minutes selecting a healthcare provider for her pregnancy. Most people spend many hours making selections on new computers or car purchases, but very little time selecting the people who support their health. Honor this selection as important to you and your baby for your family's long-term health.

Pregnancy and birth are one of the only times in your life that you will seek medical care when you are not sick. Pregnancy is not an illness, so the care that you receive during pregnancy and birth should be empowering and supportive. Seeking providers that see pregnancy as a time of health instead of a time of risk can change your entire experience. Your healthcare team includes everyone who will offer support to you throughout pregnancy. This includes the office staff, nurses, lab technicians, and of course your primary care provider—your doctor or your midwife. Often, healthcare providers work in large groups where there are several doctors or midwives, and you will see more than one provider throughout your pregnancy. If you select a group practice, it is important that you feel comfortable with *all* of the providers who are working together since they usually share on-call times, and you often cannot select who will actually be at your baby's birth.

If at any time you start to feel that you are not in conscious agreement with your healthcare team, it is important to have open communication with them about your concerns and/or change healthcare providers. Ultimately, you are the one who chooses your support team. If you find that there are major differences in your vision for your birth and your caregiver's practice, then you may want to consider seeking out a new provider with whom you can be in conscious agreement.

Additionally, your healthcare team may include some of the following types of healthcare providers:

Special Note:

A physician is a care provider who specializes in the medical support of pregnancy and childbirth. Though physicians are the most common healthcare providers in the United States, another safe option is the midwifery model of care. The midwifery model of care is a specialty that focuses on wellness through holistic healthcare management for women throughout their life cycle. If you are considering a home birth, waterbirth or unmedicated birth, a midwifery model of care may be your best option. In fact, the midwifery model may appeal to you even if you plan a hospital birth, or want to use medication for pain management.

Birthing options and place of birth will be covered in Part Four of this book. It is very important to explore your options for place of birth and types of providers very early in your pregnancy.

Obstetrician(OB)/Gynecologist: A physician/surgeon who specializes in pregnancy, labor, and postpartum medical care. Their focus is the medical management of pregnancy and birth.

High Risk OB/Specialty OB/Perinatologist: A physician/surgeon who specializes in the management of healthcare for high-risk pregnancies. Examples include: twins/triplets, fertility treatment, and certain pregnancy-related medical conditions.

Family Practice Physician: A physician who specializes in the general healthcare of the family. Not all family practice physicians provide maternity care.

Nurse Practitioner: An advanced practice nurse with a masters or doctoral degree in healthcare. Their primary focus is prevention, wellness, and education.

Certified Midwife (CM): A midwife with an approved certification from the American College of Nurse-Midwives.

Certified Nurse-Midwife (CNM): A nurse who specializes in midwifery care with an approved certification from the American College of Nurse-Midwives. CNMs, depending on the state, practice in a hospital, birth center, or homebirth setting.

Certified Professional Midwife (CPM): A midwife who specializes and is certified in midwifery care according to the North American Registry of Midwives (NARM).

Direct-Entry Midwife (DEM): A midwife who has obtained her education through apprenticeship, a midwifery school, a college program, or self-study modules. Most DEMs practice in a homebirth setting.

Lay Midwife: A midwife who has obtained education via self-study or apprenticeship. They are not certified or licensed, though may have a high level of midwifery skill.

Naturopathic Obstetrician: A holistic physician whose focus is on the wellness model of care. They have been specifically trained in the management of pregnancy, birth, and postpartum care.

Special Note:

The word doula traditionally means support person. These professionals offer a high level of non-medical specialized support to the pregnant mother and her new family. Doulas may or may not be professionally trained or certified. An in-depth interview with your prospective doula is recommended to ensure that your doula is a good match for you and your family.

Antepartum Doula: A support professional who assists pregnant women who are experiencing a high-risk pregnancy, are on bed rest, or who have certain medical conditions requiring the need for additional support during pregnancy.

Birth/Labor Doula: A professional who supports a mother/family before, during, and just after childbirth. A birth/labor doula will offer informational, physical, and emotional support. They offer continuous and uninterrupted care during labor and birth. Studies show that women who have doula support have better birth, postpartum, and breastfeeding outcomes.

Postpartum Doula: A professional who offers physical, emotional, and practical support for the new family during the first weeks of a newborn's life. Common support may include education regarding the newborn's care, breastfeeding support, meal preparation, and light household chores.

Childbirth Educator: An education specialist who offers classes/instruction for the mother and her partner on topics related to pregnancy, birth, breastfeeding, and the care of a newborn. Special classes may be available for adolescent mothers, women who want a vaginal birth after cesarean (VBAC), older siblings, and grandparents. Childbirth educators may or may not be professionally trained or certified.

Nutritionist/Dietician: A professional who offers education regarding nutrition. Nutritionists and dieticians focus on good health through balanced food choices. They can be particularly helpful for pregnant mothers who have gestational diabetes, need support in weight management, or who want to improve their overall nutrition.

Chiropractor: A licensed doctor who specializes in the manipulation of the spine, joints, and soft tissues. Often chiropractors work in a holistic setting and some can offer nutritional support, massage, acupuncture, and lifestyle counseling. Some also practice energy medicine. Many chiropractors are trained in the Webster Technique, which can be used to encourage babies in the breech or posterior position to turn in the womb. Pregnant women who experience pelvic or back pain can often find relief with chiropractic care.

Acupuncturist: A licensed, holistic medical professional who specializes in the movement of chi (energy flow meridians) through the placement of small needles and/or through acupressure. Acupuncturists often do nutritional/energy counseling and some specialize in the use of Chinese herbs. Acupuncturists are often helpful with fertility issues, with specific medical conditions related to pregnancy, with pain during pregnancy, as well as with encouraging labor to start.

Massage Therapist: A professional who offers massage therapy. They may or may not be licensed and/or certified. These specialists are particularly useful during pregnancy to help with pain management, relaxation, stress relief, and to encourage good circulation. Some massage therapists specialize in pregnancy and infant massage.

Part Two
Activities For Observing

Interviewing Healthcare Providers

Although you may not be able to hand pick every healthcare team member at all times, you do have the responsibility to choose your main healthcare providers wisely, and with conscious agreement. To determine if you are in conscious agreement with your healthcare provider, take the time to ask yourself and your care provider some questions.

Questions to ask yourself about this healthcare provider

- How do I feel about the care provider's bedside manner?
- Does she smile?
- Is she warm?
- Do I feel comfortable with her?
- Does she patiently respond to all of my questions?
- Does she seem well-informed and up-to-date in her thinking?
- Does she ask me how I feel about things?

- Does she seem to be respectful of my time?
- Do I feel cared for by the nurses and other staff at this practice?

Questions to ask the doctor

- What is your personal birth philosophy?
- Who are your back-up doctors/midwives? Can I meet them before the birth?
- If the practice has multiple doctors on staff, what determines who will be present at my birth? Will other practitioners honor the agreements that are made between us prior to birth?
- How long have you been in practice?
- Are you open to my using the services of a doula for my birth? What has your experience been with doulas?
- Does your practice have a policy regarding inductions and estimated due dates? What do you consider overdue?
- Can you briefly describe situations in which you feel cesarean birth is necessary? Can you share with me how you use instrumental delivery (forceps/vacuum delivery) and episiotomy?
- Do you feel comfortable in supporting me in any safe manner in which I choose to labor and give birth (unmedicated or natural childbirth, hypnotherapy, use of tub or shower, position of my choice, mobility during labor, epidural)?
- Does your practice specialize in high-risk or low-risk pregnancies? What do you consider a high-risk pregnancy? Does the age of the mother determine risk status?
- Does your practice work with my insurance company and/or offer payment plans for cash payment?
- What is your standard care for babies in the breech position?

- Do you support mothers who wish to have a vaginal birth after cesarean (VBAC)?
- What is the best way for me to communicate my needs/desires with you regarding my pregnancy and birth? (A birth plan, direct communication, email, etc.)
- Do you support my use of photography and/or video recording of my labor and birth? What if I have a cesarean?
- Can you share with me your philosophy about breastfeeding, skin-to-skin and bonding in the first hour and days? What specific support will you and your staff be able to provide me with in terms of breastfeeding my baby?

Questions to ask the midwife

- What is your personal birth philosophy?
- Who are your back-up doctors/midwives? Can I meet them before the birth?
- What is your training/certification/licensure? How long have you been practicing?
- Can you provide me with a list of references?
- Are you open to my using the services of a doula for my birth? What has your experience been with doulas?
- In what specific situations would my pregnancy be considered too high-risk for your care? Do you have a specific doctor you refer to in those situations? Do you attend breech birth, twin birth, VBAC birth?
- Does your practice work with my insurance company and/or offer payment plans for cash payment? What is your fee structure? If I have a homebirth and am transferred to the hospital, how does that change my payment?
- If I am having a homebirth, what safety precautions do you have in place in case of an emergency? Do you have specialized neonatal support training? What is your

relationship with the hospital I would be transferred to in the case of an emergency?

- If I am having a homebirth, what supplies do you expect me to purchase/provide? What equipment/supplies do you bring to the birth?
- How do I ensure that you will be present at my birth? What happens if you are ill or away?
- Do you offer water birth services? Do you rent water birth tubs?
- How long do you spend with me during prenatal visits?
- During a home birth, when do you come to my home during labor? If I have a hospital/birth center birth, when are you present at my labor/birth?
- How do you handle emergencies? What is your transfer rate (what percentage of the births that you attend transfer to the hospital)? In the event of a transfer, do you stay with me at the hospital?
- What care do you provide to the baby after birth? How long do you stay with me after the birth?
- What type of postpartum care do I receive after the birth?
- Can you share with me your philosophy about breast-feeding, skin-to-skin and bonding in the first hour and days? What specific support will you be able to provide me with in terms of breastfeeding my baby?

Questions to ask the doula

- What is your personal philosophy of birth?
- Do you have a backup doula? Can I meet her or interview her over the phone before the birth?
- What type of training and/or certifications do you have? How long have you been practicing? What is the best

way for me to verify your certification and references?

- How many births have you attended? What types of births have you attended?
- How do I ensure that you will be available when I go into labor?
- How many clients do you have at any one time?
- Can you explain your role as my doula at my birth?
- Are you willing to support any choice I make during my birth? Are you able to put your personal belief systems aside at my birth?
- What is your relationship like with my care provider? Are you welcomed at my birth facility?
- What are your fees? How do I make payments? What is your refund policy? What specific support do you offer to my partner?
- Do you have a contract that spells out exactly what you offer to birthing families? For example, how often will you meet with me prenatally and during the postpartum period?
- Do you have a list of resources that will be helpful to me during pregnancy and postpartum?
- When do I call you when I am in labor? How long do you stay with me after birth?
- Do you offer any additional services, such as childbirth education, belly casting, breastfeeding support, or post-partum doula care?

Medical Tests in Pregnancy and Conscious Agreement

When using conscious agreement for decisions about prenatal testing, remember that the goal is to be in conscious agreement with yourself AND your baby. Here are some general questions to ask yourself to help you decide if prenatal testing feels right:

- Is there a benefit to my baby? To myself?
- Is there a risk to my baby? To myself?
- How does having this test make me feel?
- Are the results of this particular test very accurate or do they have a high false-positive rate?
- Does the knowledge about the results change my relationship with my baby? Do I want it to? Can it help me/my baby in any way?
- Will the knowledge this test provides alter the outcome of my pregnancy? Would I change anything about my care, care provider, place of birth, or birth plan depending on the results?
- Can the diagnosis/disease this test screens for be treated effectively during/after pregnancy?
- Do I feel pressured to have the test? Is that impacting my decision?
- Are there any alternatives to the test?
- Am I in a high-risk category? Does that change my decision to have the test?
- Am I making my decision from a place of fear or a place of trust?
- What am I specifically afraid of? How might I handle the situation if my fears were realized?
- Would I feel better knowing the results?
- Is not knowing whether my child has the specific condition to be tested for affecting my ability to bond with my baby?

Typical Medical Tests Given to Pregnant Women

MEDICAL TEST
Alpha Fetoprotein, AFP

WHEN GIVEN
15-20 weeks of pregnancy

HOW ADMINISTERED
Blood test. If testing for Down syndrome, this test is combined with an ultrasound to look at the thickness of the baby's neck.

WHY
To screen for certain birth defects such as spina bifida, Down syndrome, anencephaly, Edwards syndrome, and other chromosomal anomalies by looking at the levels of alpha-fetoprotein (AFP), human chorionic gonadotropin (hCG), and estriol (uE3) in mother's blood stream.

CONSCIOUS AGREEMENT CONSIDERATIONS
Screening on average can only detect 60% of babies with Down syndrome and 80+% of babies with neural tube defects.
There is a high false positive rate, dependant on many factors. A positive screen can result in further testing, such as amniocentesis.

MEDICAL TEST
Amniocentesis

WHEN GIVEN
15-18 weeks of pregnancy

HOW ADMINISTERED
A mother lies down and ultrasound is performed to determine where the baby is lying in the womb. A needle is inserted from the external abdomen to inside the womb where amniotic fluid can be drawn. The amniotic fluid is then tested as it contains genetic material from the baby.

WHY

Used to detect Down syndrome, spina bifida and neural tube defects, sickle cell disease, cystic fibrosis, muscular dystrophy and Tay Sachs disease.

CONSCIOUS AGREEMENT CONSIDERATIONS
Babies have been shown to experience high levels of stress during this test. Their heart rates become elevated, and they sometimes bat or kick at the amniocentesis needle. The baby's level of cortisol or stress hormone increases. Amniocentesis increases risk of miscarriage, cramping, bleeding and infection.

MEDICAL TEST
Blood Draw

WHEN GIVEN
Throughout pregnancy, at prenatal visits

HOW ADMINISTERED
Use needle to draw blood from a vein.

WHY
Done initially to confirm pregnancy and to determine blood type and rhesus status. Can also be used for disease screening, such as HIV, rubella, syphilis, and hepatitis B. It can also be done to determine if you are anemic or if you are diabetic.

CONSCIOUS AGREEMENT CONSIDERATIONS
If you're Rh-negative, you'll get a shot of Rh immunoglobulin at least once during your pregnancy, as well as after delivery if your baby turns out to be Rh-positive. This shot will protect you from developing antibodies that could be dangerous during this pregnancy or in future pregnancies. (Note: If your baby's father is also Rh-negative, your baby will be too, so you won't need the shot.)

MEDICAL TEST
Blood Pressure

WHEN GIVEN
At prenatal visits and periodically during labor and birth.

HOW ADMINISTERED
A cuff is placed around your upper arm. Air is forced into the cuff. A stethoscope is used to listen to your pulse as the blood pressure cuff takes the reading.

WHY
Can determine if you have high or low blood pressure.

CONSCIOUS AGREEMENT CONSIDERATIONS
Your blood pressure is strongly affected by your emotional state and your state of anxiety. Try to take a few moments to close your eyes and use deep breathing techniques prior to having your blood pressure read. Some women tend to get nervous at their care providers office, which can elevate the blood pressure.

MEDICAL TEST
Chorionic Villus Sampling, CVS

WHEN GIVEN
10-12 weeks

HOW ADMINISTERED
The removal of a small piece of chorionic villus which contains genetic material similar to your baby either via a needle placed through the abdomen into the uterus or through a catheter placed in the vagina through the cervix and into the placenta. Ultrasound is used to determine placement of baby and placenta.

WHY
Use to predict Down syndrome, Tay Sachs and over 200 other genetic disorders or chromosomal birth defects. Can be done earlier than amniocentesis. Can also be done to determine blood type if Rh sensitization has occurred.

CONSCIOUS AGREEMENT CONSIDERATIONS
Can increase the risk of bleeding, miscarriage, infection, rupture of membranes, Rh sensitization. Can increase risk of breathing difficulties for babies at birth and also increases risk of club-foot.

MEDICAL TEST
External Fetal Heart Monitoring

WHEN GIVEN
Throughout pregnancy and during labor and birth

HOW ADMINISTERED
Ultrasound technology that involves placing electrodes on the mother's abdomen over a conducting gel which sense the baby's heartbeat.

WHY
Used to determine the heart rate of the baby, which can be an indicator of health and stress level.

CONSCIOUS AGREEMENT CONSIDERATIONS
The external monitor is not always entirely accurate as the reading of the results is determined by the training and observation of the healthcare provider. Research shows that healthcare practitioners vary widely in their diagnosis of heart monitor samplings.

MEDICAL TEST
Nuchal Translucency Screening

WHEN GIVEN
11-14 weeks

HOW ADMINISTERED
An ultrasound exam is performed to check the thickness of the back of the baby's neck. They also test your blood for levels of a protein called pregnancy-associated plasma protein and a hormone called human chorionic gonadotropin (hCG).

WHY
To determine birth defects such as Down syndrome, Turner syndrome, Trisomy 18 and Trisomy 13, as well as other chromosomal abnormalities. It can also be used to check pregnancy dates and the viability of the pregnancy.

CONSCIOUS AGREEMENT CONSIDERATIONS
There is no evidence on the safety of nuchal scans, nor if they are more effective than traditional scans. Effectiveness rates range from 60-80% and false positive rate can be as high as 5%.

MEDICAL TEST
Transvaginal Scan

WHEN GIVEN
Throughout pregnancy

HOW ADMINISTERED
An ultrasound probe is inserted into the vagina to look at the baby, placenta, etc. It is closer to the womb and allows ultrasonic waves to be more accurate.

WHY
Used to assess health status of baby, pregnancy dates, health of placenta and a variety of other screening tests.

CONSCIOUS AGREEMENT CONSIDERATIONS
Because the ultrasonic waves do not have to go through the abdominal muscles and fat the level of ultrasound on your baby is greater. See ultrasound.

MEDICAL TEST
Ultrasound

WHEN GIVEN
Throughout pregnancy and during labor and birth

HOW ADMINISTERED
High frequency sound waves are bounced off the baby and placenta to get a view of inside the womb.

WHY
Used to assess health status of baby, pregnancy dates, health of placenta and a variety of other screening tests.

CONSCIOUS AGREEMENT CONSIDERATIONS
The long-term effects of ultrasound are still unclear, though it is known that heat and cavitation does occur (vapor bubbles occurring in cells and amniotic fluid). Additionally, it may alter brain function, damage soft tissues and slightly increase the risk of miscarriage.

MEDICAL TEST
Urine test

WHEN GIVEN
Throughout pregnancy and during labor

HOW ADMINISTERED
Mother provides a urine sample in a cup. A dip-stick is often inserted to test certain conditions.

WHY
Can be used to confirm pregnancy. Also used to see if protein is in the urine, a condition called pre-eclampsia. Can be used to look for infection, as well.

Part Two:
Keynotes For Observing

The way that you observe your world will influence your pregnancy and your baby's health.

Reducing stress is key to a happier, healthier pregnancy and baby. Commit yourself to reducing stressful situations in your life and when experiencing stress, practice the following:

- Use the Four A's: Avoid, Alter, Adapt and Accept
- Deep breathing activities
- Smiling and laughing
- Yawning
- Focusing on your heart space

Healthy nutrition includes eating clean and natural, enjoy healthy oils, noshing on veggies, finding good sources of vitamins and minerals, avoiding no-value foods and moving your body.

Focus on your most supportive relationships during pregnancy. Consciously create your circles of support. Decide who belongs in your inner circle and who belongs in your outer circles.

When it is time to select your healthcare providers and decide on medical tests in pregnancy, remember to use conscious agreement.

Part Three

The Second Trimester of Pregnancy

B-O-*N*-D
N stands for Nourish

"When you recover or discover something that nourishes your soul and brings you joy, care enough about yourself to make room for it in your life."
—Jean Shinoda Bolen

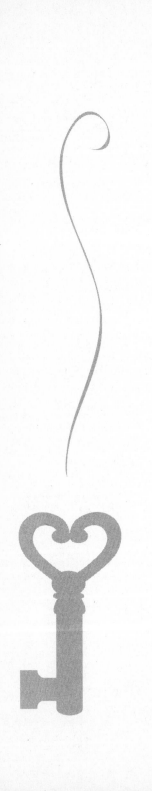

Chapter Ten

Nourishing Yourself and Your Baby

"Why are we here? We exist not to pursue happiness, which is fleeting, or outer accomplishment, which can always be bettered. We are here to nourish the self."
—Deepak Chopra

The motherbaby bond is cultivated early in your pregnancy as you nourish your mind, body, and spirit. Your intentions, actions, and who and how you love play a vital role in your baby's development in the second trimester. Your baby's sensory organs begin to develop, along with her awareness of the world that lies outside the womb. During the second trimester, everything you experience in your world will form what your baby knows of the world. Your baby shares the flavors of food you taste, the sound of the music you listen to, and the feelings of love you have for her and others in your life. This early relationship between you and your child will be the first guiding map for your baby to navigate her emotional world.

When you choose a nourishing environment for yourself, it also enriches your baby's world. Even at this early stage, your baby is conscious and responding to love, or a lack thereof. The second trimester is often when you begin to feel not only an emotional connection but a physical connection to your baby; these first movements you feel in the womb are sometimes called quickening. Your baby begins to respond to sounds, movement, voices, and your emotions by crying, smiling, and thumb sucking. Your baby already has a profound emotional life well before she is born. The miracle of the motherbaby bond unfolds and deepens during the second trimester, as your heart, mind, and body constantly communicate with your baby.

What's Up, Baby?

Weeks 13–16: Lanugo, a fine hair, begins to develop on your baby's body. Your baby's bones and muscle tissue begin to develop. By 15 weeks the development of the external genitals is complete. Though your baby's vision is limited, it is functional at this stage. Your baby's sense of touch becomes more refined. Your baby uses her hands to interact with her environment, including the umbilical cord, her mouth, or her twin brother or sister. Taste buds are developed by week 14, and it is believed that babies can taste at this stage. Your baby will gulp faster with sweet flavors in the amniotic fluid (from the foods you eat) and she swallows more slowly when there are bitter or sour flavors present. Your baby's sense of smell is functioning, and though your baby "smells" in a different way than she will when she is born, she experiences up to 120 different smell compounds. By week 16, reactive listening begins, before the ear has even completed its development. This means your baby reacts to sounds outside the womb.

Weeks 16–20: Your baby grows to be about 9 inches long from head to feet. She has eyelashes and eyebrows. You may feel quickening around 16 weeks, or the first movement of your baby inside you. Her sense of vision is developing. Twins have been observed kissing and stroking one another at this stage.

Weeks 20–24: Your baby's finger and footprints are developing. Her lungs begin to mature. Her ear structure is complete. The most important sound to your baby is the sound of your voice.

Your baby responds to sounds outside the womb and reacts to those sounds. Your baby learns about the people in your life based on these sounds and the emotional molecules that you share with her. She will know the people in your life long before she is born.

Weeks 24–27: Your baby grows to be about 15 inches long from head to foot and weighs about 2 pounds, 11 ounces. Her eyelids begin to open. Her respiratory system has developed enough to allow for gas exchange and her lungs are beginning to produce surfactant, a substance that will help her breathe when she is born. She begins to inhale and exhale the surrounding amniotic fluid to prepare for breathing at birth. Her sense of balance and position is complete. Her taste buds are refining and your baby's palate is expanding based on the flavors in the amniotic fluid, which change depending on your diet. This is also the age when your baby will start growing hair on her head. She will also begin to sleep and wake in regular patterns.

What's Up, Mama?

By now you may start to feel more energy and be less nauseous. This is an exciting time, especially as you begin to feel your baby move inside of you. Most women report feeling their baby moving between 16–19 weeks. The first movements sometimes feel like a fluttering sensation. If you choose to learn the sex of your baby, an ultrasound can often determine your baby's gender during this time. A dark line may appear from your navel down to your pubic area; this is called the linea nigra, and it will fade away after shortly after birth. It may become more difficult to catch your breath as your uterus grows and expands into the abdomen. You may also feel a sense of relief knowing that the chances of miscarriage are significantly reduced at this stage. Your libido may increase and intercourse can be very enjoyable during the second trimester. It's common to see some stretch marks as your skin begins to stretch to accommodate your growing baby and breasts. Your breasts begin to prepare to feed your baby by making colostrum, your baby's first milk. You may begin to feel some of the common discomforts of pregnancy such as pelvic pressure, backache, and heartburn during this trimester. You may find yourself waking frequently to urinate as your baby and uterus grow and put pressure on the bladder. Your hair and fingernails grow faster and may seem healthier. This is a great time to keep your body healthy by continuing or starting a daily exercise regimen like walking, prenatal yoga, or swimming.

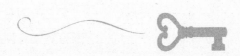

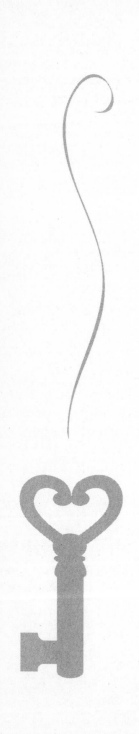

Chapter Eleven

*Keys to Giving
and Receiving Love*

"Love is the capacity to take care, to protect, to nourish. If you are not capable of generating that kind of energy toward yourself- if you are not capable of taking care of yourself, of nourishing yourself, of protecting yourself- it is very difficult to take care of another person... it's clear that to love oneself is the foundation of the love of other people. Love is a practice. Love is truly a practice."
—**Thich Nhat Hanh**

During the second trimester, your baby is developing the foundation for her emotional life. Every thought you have and every emotion you feel is communicated directly to your baby. She begins to understand the world outside based on what your emotions communicate to her. This prenatal period has the most impact on her emotional health because your baby's emotional center in the brain develops during this trimester.

In addition to the development of the lobes of your baby's brain, the brain wave activity is also undergoing development. During pregnancy your baby's brain is in the delta brain wave mode. This mode is one of deep sleep and regeneration, and it is in this brain wave pattern that humans report experiencing the deepest connection to their source and the collective unconscious. This developmental period is one where your baby is in a constant state of feeling. You, as a mother, have a lot of creative power during this time to offer the deepest love and joy to your baby.

The delta brain phase connects your baby to her subconscious mind. This is the part of mind that will form your baby's habits and core beliefs about the world. The subconscious mind will rule her behavior and the majority of her thoughts for life. The subconscious always functions in the present tense, meaning that the subconscious mind cannot differentiate experiences in the past from experiences in the present. This means your baby's emotional experience during your pregnancy, as her subconscious mind is forming, will be the emotional story her mind tells her over and over again for the rest of her life. As a mother, you have the power to write this beginning chapter of her story, and to make it a happy tale.

The subconscious mind is formed based on emotional states, not intellectual thought. It is the mind of emotions and feeling. If your baby has a prenatal experience filled primarily with stress and anxiety, her brain is set to expect anxiety and stress throughout her life. Alternatively, if she often experiences rushes of love and joy hormones, her mind is set to anticipate love in her world. Every experience your baby has during the prenatal period forms the foundation for all she perceives about the world. You love your baby and you want her to have a positive outlook on life, have healthy relationships, be loving and kind, and enjoy life. Pregnancy and the first years of your baby's life will be the most influential time when you can invest in who your child will become and what her world-view will be.

Your baby's brain, though still very immature, is developing at astounding rates during the second trimester. At this point in your baby's life, her brain changes based on environmental factors that you are exposed to. Every experience your child has in the womb changes the wiring of your baby's brain. Dr. Joe Dispenza, who wrote the book *Evolve Your Brain*, often says "what fires together, wires together." This means that the more you experience an emotion or situation, the more your brain is designed to expect that emotion or situation. You can help design your child's brain to form a positive mental attitude by engaging in positive emotions yourself. What an amazing gift to give your child!

⚷ Master Keys – Tips From the Experts

The following is an excerpt from an interview with international neuroscience expert and author, Dr. Joe Dispenza. Dr. Dispenza was featured in the hit movie What the Bleep Do We Know!? and is the author of the book Evolve Your Brain: The Science of Changing Your Mind.

"It's a scientific fact that 95 percent of who we are is the subconscious mind and it's made up of our habits, our behaviors, our skills, and emotional reactions. The conscious mind is made up of logic and reasoning which gives way to our willpower and our creative abilities. In utero, all of the information that a baby perceives is based on her internal state. It is derived primarily from how she feels, and it is encoded directly into the subconscious mind. The experience in utero begins to write the script for some of those unconscious behaviors that will surface later on in life when the child is experiencing those same conditions.

Bonding is a very mid-brain function, a subconscious function. Bonding is based on feelings; it's based on sharing emotions. If you share the same emotions, you share the same energy. If you share the same energy, you are functioning as a whole. When you're functioning in wholeness, because you're exchanging that information energetically, that wholeness is a very strong foundation to build from.

One of the strongest bonds that we have in the human species is the connection between a mother and a child. When a mother gets her values right…there is a very innate way in which she begins to change her priorities. That means she begins to make choices for the long term health of her child: taking time alone, in meditation, in reading, in expressing love instead of fear, in telling the truth, in bonding with other women that are pregnant who are working towards the same ideals and goals, taking time to rest and sleep. All of these instinctual things create a growth and repair state. There is a knowing that happens. They just have to trust and listen to it."

More on Stress in Pregnancy

The emotions your baby experiences during pregnancy begin the intricate wiring of her brain. This is how the human brain adapts itself for survival outside the womb; your baby is in constant preparation for the world she will encounter when she is born. Studies have shown that the prenatal experience impacts your baby's brain size, her ability to reason later in life, and can even determine when she is born.

There is a well-known study called the Hongerwinter study, which studied the children born to the women who experienced the Dutch famine of 1944. During this time, the Netherlands was occupied by the Nazis and nearly 18,000 people died of starvation. Women who were pregnant during this period experienced terribly high levels of stress and starvation. Researchers were surprised to learn that not only were the babies born to these women smaller, but these children's future babies were also smaller. The experience in the womb actually changed the genetic expression of the babies, meaning their physical and mental health was altered. Additionally, these children were more likely to experience schizophrenia, bipolar disorder, and other mental disorders directly related to the high levels of stress. During pregnancy, their brains became conditioned to expect the world to be a stressful and scary place.

This study's results have been replicated many times over in different cultures throughout our recent history. There is a definitive link between high levels of stress in pregnancy and alterations in the baby's brain chemistry and genetic expression. Studies have looked at babies born during China's Great Leap Forward, the Iraq War, Children of the 90's (in Avon, England), and children in utero during the attacks on the U.S. on September 11, 2001. Each of these studies had similar results: when pregnant women experienced high stress levels, their babies were impacted. These studies showed a variety of effects that included, but were not limited to, premature birth, changes in brain chemistry and mental health, and increased risk of heart disease. Babies are not shielded from their mother's stress; they take it as a cue for what their future has in store for them. Babies begin to prepare for that future while they are still in the womb. While it is unlikely that you will experience a stressor such as the terrible events mentioned, you still might be in a state of chronic stress. Pregnant women are often in chronic states of stress due to today's high-paced, output focused, high demand society.

The first part of your baby's brain to develop is the limbic system, which includes the amygdala and hippocampus, also known as the primitive brain regions. These parts of the brain activate our "gut reactions" and are intrinsic to human survival. The primitive brain processes memory, emotion, and reactions to stress. Chronic stress in a mother can alter the healthy development of these parts of the brain in her baby.

It is important to pay attention to how you are feeling and how your body is reacting to life's stressors so that you can help your baby develop a healthy, strong brain that is wired with many positive neural connections. This early brain development is critical for creating your baby's emotional experiences and serves as the conductor of your child's emotional "choir." Every emotional response to the world is directed by this primitive part of her brain.

The human capacity to love, both giving and receiving, is something that only develops from the time of conception through the toddler years. If humans do not experience love during their formative years, the life-long results are detrimental and irreversible. In fact, the most basic need for human babies, stronger even than the need for food, is the need to be loved. Some studies have shown that baby mammals will ignore food to receive love. Love is vital to growth. Creating healthy love connections for your child prenatally is easy: send her love!

The late Dr. Frederick Wirth, a neonatologist who cared for the first test tube baby in the United States, was the pioneer of the course Prenatal Parenting™. Dr. Wirth's course was developed for expectant families to help them bond with their babies before birth. During his life, he lectured extensively on the importance of loving yourself, your baby, and your partner for optimal development of your baby. While caring for the most fragile babies in the neonatal intensive care unit, he began studying the impact of the prenatal environment on the baby. He quickly realized that the baby was impacted significantly by the mother's emotional state. It became his mission in life to help educate families on the importance of this prenatal period. He taught families how to use "Fetal Love Breaks" throughout the day as a means of forming a deep bond between mother and baby. Fetal Love Breaks are easy to do, and better yet, they take very little time. His concept simply involved closing your eyes and for several minutes sending your baby loving messages. You can do this anywhere, anytime.

Part of the reason Fetal Love Breaks work is that when you are experiencing the emotion of love your brain is releasing the hormone oxytocin. Oxytocin is known as the bonding or love hormone. Humans release this hormone at critical bonding moments: falling in love, experiencing loving touch, experiencing orgasm, giving birth, breastfeeding, and simply by being present and connected to those you love. This hormone excites the part of the brain that creates attachment. The flood of oxytocin you feel at these moments affects the emotional center of the brain and you experience it as the feeling of love. The more your baby experiences oxytocin rushes from your loving thoughts during pregnancy, the more her brain becomes wired to expect, desire, and reciprocate love. This is how very early attachment occurs. Before your baby is born, you are creating attachments. Dr. Wirth called this "becoming a brain architect."

Interestingly, researchers have discovered that your baby communicates back to you. When your baby experiences emotions, her emotional states are communicated back to you via a series of complex hormonal reactions through the umbilical cord and placenta. The two of you share an emotional experience. The more you send love to your baby, the more she sends love back to you. Alternatively, your baby also can feel your fears, anger, and anxieties. Don't let this worry you too much. In fact, allowing yourself to have a healthy array of emotions helps your child to create emotional intelligence (EQ which stands for emotional quotient). Babies should experience the full range of your emotions in pregnancy for optimal health. In fact, when babies experience short-term stress in the womb, they learn to become stress hardy. It is only when stress is chronic and unrelenting that it has a negative effect on your baby. Stress is normal, it is natural, and it is a healthy part of pregnancy. However, the human body most effectively deals with stress that is short-lived, not chronic.

The key to creating a healthy EQ in your baby is to allow yourself to fully experience your emotions, and then, if it is not an emotion that nourishes you and your baby, release it. Here are some easy ways to return your mind to a peaceful state after experiencing a stressful event:

- Close your eyes and take a few deep breaths. Practice deep breathing techniques. Breath is known in eastern cultures as prana, or the life force. Connecting to that life force can have life sustaining benefits including helping you to release stress. To "inspire" means to breathe in. Use your breath to inspire you towards a deeper connection with your baby, towards a state of peace. Breathing in and out through your nose also has added benefit of lowering anxiety.

- Move into breathing awareness and think about something that pleases you. Bring your attention to the area around your heart and connect with the energy in your heart. Stay focused there until you begin to feel balanced. It is helpful to actually place one hand over your heart and one hand on your belly. You can also focus on a word, a phrase, or a chant that feels supportive, calming, or peaceful to you.

- Yawn. It sounds strange, but yawning has enormous health benefits. In the book *How God Changes Your Brain: Breakthrough Findings from a Leading Neuroscientist*, by Newman and Waldman, the authors discuss how yawning can calm the mind in less than a minute. They recommend practicing yawning at least 12–15 times, pausing for a few seconds between each yawn. If you find it challenging, just fake yawn until real yawning begins. The authors state that yawning stimulates a part of the brain called the precuneous, which is partly responsible for feelings of empathy, consciousness, and self-awareness. Yawning helps you reset and stabilize your mind. So give it a go, sit back, relax, and yawn. (Interestingly, it is during the second trimester that your baby begins to yawn!)

Fathers and partners are not left out of the love equation. Your relationship with your primary partner during pregnancy has a significant impact on your child. During the second trimester, your baby can hear and she begins to associate the voice of your partner with the emotions you experience when around him or her. Your child starts to have a relationship with her father (or your partner) well before she is born. There are ultrasounds that have shown a baby crying in the womb after an explosive fight between his mother and father. Ultrasounds have also shown babies smiling, grimacing, and showing body movements that indicate protection. It was once believed that these were simply reflexes of the baby and that they had no relationship to a baby's real emotional experience. It is now known that babies have a rich emotional life in the womb and they react physically and emotionally to their experiences.

So what does this mean about your relationship with your partner? It means there is no better time than time than now to develop a more loving, communicative, and deep relationship with the person who will be parenting with you.

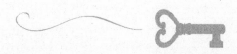

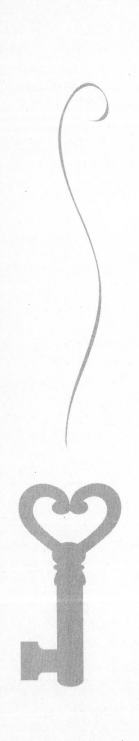

Chapter Twelve

*Keys to a Nourishing
Partner Relationship*

*"Even after all this time, the sun never says to the Earth, 'you owe
me.' Look what happens with a love like that, it lights the whole sky."*
—**Hafiz**

---

*Note from the authors: While we realize and honor the fact that not every
pregnant woman has a partner, nor is every partner a man, we have chosen
to use the terms father/partner/dad to describe the partner relationship. While
some of the information in this chapter is specifically written for the father/
male, much of it can be applied to other relationships, such as same sex partners or single mothers who have a mother/sister/friend in a supportive role.*

Pregnancy will bring changes to your relationship that start now and
that continue as your family grows. It is very normal in pregnancy to
have moments that you are excited as well as times when you question
what you have gotten yourself into. Your feelings and your acceptance
of your partner's feelings can strengthen your relationship or place a
strain on it. Pregnancy is a time of rapid emotional and physical change.
Loving communication with your partner is crucial during this time.

During the second trimester, your baby can hear your voice in utero as well as the voice of your partner. Being consciously aware of your communication as a couple and expressing loving gratitude towards each other is far more important than you may think. Remember that your baby is a feeling person, and your baby feels your emotions. Your growing and developing baby is directly affected by the relationship you and your partner have with one another. Your baby will recognize you both at birth because her relationship with both of you has been forming throughout pregnancy. Practicing loving and grateful communication before birth only strengthens your family and builds a strong foundation for parenting after birth. The parental relationship is the first relationship most children observe and learn from. They learn to love by observing their parents' relationship. Children from families whose parents have a loving and nourishing relationship feel safer and more secure in their world.

Looking at Your Relationship

Does the relationship you have with your partner nourish you? Does your partner feel nourished in your relationship? The components of a nourishing relationship include both the giving and receiving of love, care, and positive communication. Just like an untended garden, when relationships aren't nourished and tended to, you cannot expect an abundant and plentiful harvest. People need attention and love, and when these aspects of a relationship are not protected, relationships wither.

Often relationships start down the road to neglect simply because life takes over and attentions become scattered. In today's world you may feel pulled in a million different directions and it is easy to misdirect your attention to things that seem urgent, instead of the things that are most important. Things like work, household chores, returning calls and emails, and participating in social media are often the distractions that take time and attention away from your relationships. What are your priorities? Is time with your partner more important than watching television? If your priorities are not with your partner, this is an indication of being disconnected with yourself, your family, and your consciousness. It means you are practicing unconsciousness regarding the needs of yourself and your partner.

Moving into consciousness in your partnership means becoming aware of your relationship habits. These habits are actions you regularly do that, over time, either build your relationship or harm it. Practicing consciousness by being aware of these habits and making changes when necessary will strengthen your relationship. Even more importantly, it will strengthen your family's bond. Your relationship with your partner is no longer exclusive between the two of you, as it now involves your baby. The relationship your baby has with her father during pregnancy is literally the relationship you have with him now. Remember, your baby experiences people outside the womb, specifically her father, based on the emotional reactions you have when he is near you.

If you often harbor negative thoughts about your partner, find that you are feeling angry, experience resentment or disappointment within your relationship, now is the time to address those feelings. The longer these issues are left unchecked, the more it affects your baby's future relationship with this person and potentially your familial relationship. If changes are necessary, now is the time to make them.

Gratitude for your partner is critical to a nourishing relationship. What is it you value about this person? What positive things do they bring to your relationship? In what ways do they care for you? Dr. Gary Chapman wrote a wonderful book called *The 5 Love Languages*, which is an excellent resource to help identify the ways couples can show love for one another. His book is based on the idea that everyone has a love language, which is the way a person communicates love. Dr. Chapman states that often partners speak different love languages and, in fact, are drawn to people who speak a love language other than their own. These five languages are: words of affirmation, quality time, receiving gifts, acts of service, and physical touch.

Have you been aware of your partner's love language? Do you

express gratitude for the ways he shows he loves you? Even more critical, do you take time to *feel* gratitude for his acts of love? Begin today. Experience gratitude and love for your partner. Find at least one way your partner expresses his love and sit for a few minutes in gratitude for this act of love. Even better, tell your partner that you notice what he does for you and express your gratitude for these things to him, no matter how small.

> *Encouragement requires empathy and seeing the world from your spouse's perspective. We must first learn what is important to our spouse. Only then can we give encouragement. With verbal encouragement, we are trying to communicate, 'I know. I care. I am with you. How can I help?' We are trying to show that we believe in him and in his abilities. We are giving credit and praise.*
>
> —Dr. Gary Chapman

Partners Experience of Pregnancy

Couvade is a French term that means phantom pregnancy or sympathy pregnancy. This syndrome occurs when men experience some of the symptoms of the mother's pregnancy, including backaches, weight gain, cramping, nausea, and sensations that feel like contractions. Some men even experience postpartum depression. In a very real way, many fathers are just as "pregnant" as the mother is. However, the father's experience of the pregnancy is uniquely different.

During pregnancy, there will be times when you both feel very connected to one another, just as there will be times when you feel like you are not on the same page. This is normal and due mainly to the different ways that female and male brains are wired and the hormones their bodies produce. The female brain is designed to nurture, nourish, protect and love her baby from the moment of conception. The male brain is designed to care for his mate and develop a bond to his child once the baby is born. The hormones of pregnancy are responsible for the increased feelings of nurturing, as well as the heightened emotions of the mother. The more physically close a partner is to the mother during pregnancy, the more likely these hormones that promote bonding will be elevated in him, as well.

Mothers often express feelings of concern that the father does not share her same level of connection to the baby during pregnancy. It's very important for mothers to understand that this is normal for fathers. In fact, the father's hormones that create the bond between him and his baby are released at their *highest levels* when he is present at labor and birth, when he holds his baby and participates in caretaking activities, and when he is near the breastfeeding mother. These hormones are oxytocin and vasopressin, respectively known as the bonding and monogamy hormones. Men are designed to do the most bonding with babies after birth, not before, though many dads feel a very close bond to their child during pregnancy. You should not be alarmed if dad is not quite as excited as you are about picking out the crib or the color of the nursery. It does not mean he doesn't love you or the baby.

Today's dads' involvement in pregnancy, childbirth, and parenting has changed significantly from the previous generation. More than ninety percent of U.S. fathers are present at birth. Today's father is more likely to attend prenatal visits, go to childbirth classes, be active in selecting childcare, or even be the primary caregiver at home when the baby arrives. Fathers today are more emotionally and physically involved in their children's lives than ever before. That does not mean that their fears have disappeared.

Common concerns of expectant fathers are:

The mother's health. Your body is changing, your moods are changing, your healthcare needs are changing. He is adjusting to who you are now. Dads report that the health of their partner is one of their primary concerns during pregnancy. Like you, your partner has had a lifetime of media influences depicting the inaccurate message that pregnancy is dangerous and birth even more so. He may harbor fear about your safety during pregnancy, labor and birth.

Financial stability. Your family's financial needs have changed. This can place a strain on any relationship. Not only are there additional healthcare expenses associated with pregnancy and birth, there are additional costs to consider. These include, but are not limited to, baby gear, the possibility of new housing needs, potential need for a larger family vehicle, missed time at work, and the enormous cost of raising a child. The U.S. government currently estimates the cost to raise a child through age 17 is between $206,000 and $477,000 depending on your income bracket (not including the cost of college). Dads can become overwhelmed quickly because of their desire to provide for their family.

His ability to father/parent. Dads begin to think about what kind of father they want to be. They begin to consider their relationship with their own father, how they want to be like them, and how they want to be different. Just like you, and every other parent that has come before you, he may worry that he does not have what it takes.

The couple's sex life. Pregnancy changes your sex life. Period. Even though sex in pregnancy is generally regarded as normal, safe, and healthy, there are emotional and physical concerns for both partners. You may feel too tired, have a decreased sex drive, or be too uncomfortable to want to engage in sex. You may want to have sex, but dad may be fearful. He may have concerns about hurting the baby or hurting you. He may have an unrealistic idea of what the baby is exposed to during sex. You might be surprised to know that many dads have an unfounded fear that their penis will somehow come into contact with the baby and potentially cause harm. Taking a childbirth class together can help you both understand the anatomy of pregnancy and process of birth, as well as reduce fears around engaging in intercourse. Sometimes couples find that it takes creativity and a willingness to try many different positions and intimacy options before they find what works best in pregnancy. The hormone that is released during lovemaking is oxytocin, the love and bonding hormone. You can be comforted to know that your baby is not stressed by intercourse, in fact, she receives benefits from the oxytocin that is flowing. Go ahead. Get your groove on! If you are worried about some aspect of sex during pregnancy talk to your healthcare provider.

The change in your relationship and rituals of your relationship. Friday night date night, coffee at Starbucks, waterskiing at the lake together, sharing a glass of wine, these routines have changed and dad may now be missing his connection to you. It's normal for both of you to miss aspects of your relationship that must be temporarily put on hold. Fathers may feel even more isolated because they don't have the social perks of pregnancy. The world loves pregnant women. Dad does not have the physical proof of being an expectant dad. He is not celebrated as an expectant dad. In fact, when he is apart from you, no one is rubbing his belly or asking if he is having a boy or girl. It's no wonder that dads often feel a little left out.

Additional responsibilities. In addition to your family's financial responsibilities increasing, there are many other responsibilities that will primarily become his, including the ever-expanding honey-do list. There are simply tasks that a pregnant mom should no longer do, like cleaning a cat litter box (risk of toxoplasmosis), heavy lifting (risk of ligament injury), and painting the nursery (toxic fumes). Dads often have to work harder at their jobs because they are worried about finances and they have even less time to relax during their off time. Not only does he now have additional responsibilities during his time off, he will have even less time for the hobbies he loves, like playing video games, fishing, hanging out with his friends, working out, etc. In fact, some pastimes may be eliminated altogether due to new priorities. For example, some dads may have enjoyed motorcycle riding. This may no longer be an activity that he will participate in after the baby arrives due to a change in priorities like safety issues, available time, and cost. Not being able to participate in activities that previously brought joy is something the two of you will want to talk about it. Often new parents go through a stage of grief as they mourn the loss of their old lives. Letting go of who you both were as childless individuals can be a process. Take time to talk about ways you both can carve time into your new lives for things you *can do* and enjoy. Babies do change your life. While its true that there will be a need to let go of many things, there is the arrival of wonderful new things to come that can only be experienced as a parent, like the first time you both will hold your warm, snuggly baby against you or hear your child's laughter.

Keys to Conscious Agreement for Positive Partner Communication

Conscious awareness of your communication style with one another is important to nourishing yourself and your partner. You need to talk about your worries with one another, which means being vulnerable. This can feel very uncomfortable. However, in a truly nurturing relationship, true communication is of utmost importance. By choosing not to talk honestly with one another about your feel-ings and concerns, you are a building a wall that separates you and hinders a nourishing relationship. If you begin creating walls during pregnancy, it will be even more difficult to break down the barriers when the baby is born. The very nature of a wall means that there are two sides with a barrier in between. There is a "your" side and a "my" side, and no "our" side. Removing walls allows for "we" instead of "me." The most successful parenting involves embracing the "we" concept, as opposed to the "me" concept.

When entering into important discussions, first check in with yourself. There is a self-care technique called H.A.L.T., which can help you identify when to "halt" or stop conversations or important interaction. H.A.L.T. stands for being hungry, angry, lonely, or tired. Communicating with your partner when one, or both of you, is in a state of H.A.L.T. can lead to harmful and hurtful outcomes because your body and mind are in disconnect. When you are hungry, angry, lonely, or tired you are more likely to say things you don't mean or that are intended to cause harm. You should "halt" communication and first take care of your basic needs. Take a nap, eat a snack, or practice techniques to release stress. By practicing the self-care technique H.A.L.T. you can identify when you need to put off important and meaningful conversations. Important decisions and discussions should never be made when you are feeling hungry, angry, lonely, or tired.

Conscious agreement during communication involves being honest, truthful, and speaking from your heart. When you are using conscious agreement, you are speaking from your heart and not your ego. The ego just wants to be right, whereas the heart wants to be understood and loved.

Things to consider for communicating in conscious agreement:

You want to speak in terms of "I" not "you." For example, "I feel very lonely when you play golf on the weekends and we have so little time together" versus "You make me feel like you don't care about me when you play golf on the weekends." The first sentence identifies only your feelings. It is not accusatory. It does not put your partner immediately on the defensive.

You are responsible at all times for what you say and how you act, regardless of how others choose to engage and communicate. The old adage is true, two wrongs don't make a right. Even if you feel wounded or hurt during a conversation with your partner, it is important to not try and one up them by saying harmful things back. As soon as you behave in this manner, you have moved out of conscious agreement and moved further from the relationship that you want to have.

Stay in the present. When communicating, talk about the specific issue you want to address. Do not resort to bringing up the past or discussing "hot button" topics that you know will upset your partner.

Stay on task and be specific. Address issues as they arise, and when you can discuss them calmly. Don't let issues go unresolved, as this causes resentment.

Observe yourself when you communicate with others. Are you communicating in a manner in which you would want to be communicated to? Are you yelling, name-calling, using force, blaming, swearing, threatening to leave your partner or otherwise communicating in a destructive manner? Think about it, would you want your child to observe and emulate this behavior? Remember, your baby IS experiencing this behavior, even before she is born.

Develop your listening skills. Listening is just as much a part of communication as sharing is. True listening means that you not only hear what your partner is saying, but you also reflect back to them what you have heard. This is called *reflective listening*. Reflective listening does not require you to solve the problem or agree with your partner's point of view. It does let your partner feel validated and listened to, which is what everyone wants.

Here is an example of reflective listening:

Dad: I wish that we could have sex more often. It seems like it has been weeks.

Mom: (*not using reflective listening skills*) All you ever want to do is have sex. You don't understand how tired I am.

Instead…

Mom: (*using reflective listening skills*) I understand that you want to be more intimate, so do I. Since I am so tired this time of night, how can we compromise so that both of us can have our needs met?

Dad: (*using reflective listening skills*) Honey, I know you are really tired. How about we make a date for Saturday morning and just cuddle on the couch right now?

Using reflective listening skills can make a huge difference in all of your relationships. There are many books on reflective listening if you feel that this is a skill you wish to develop further.

The relationship you have with your partner has a very real physical and emotional impact on you and your baby. Cultivating a healthy relationship now will lead to a happier you, a happier partner, a happier baby, and ultimately a happier family.

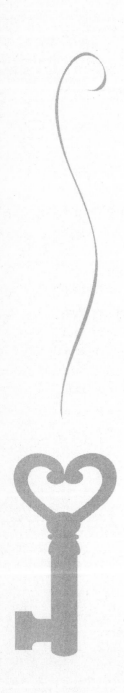

Chapter Thirteen

Keys to Physical Support in the Second Trimester

"A good laugh and a long sleep are the best cures in the doctor's book."
—Irish Proverb

Many women often feel a renewed strength in the second trimester. The body often (though not always) has adjusted to the various pregnancy hormones, and morning sickness often lessens or goes away completely. Your belly has grown large enough to make your pregnancy visible to others, but your baby is still small enough to allow for comfortable breathing, moving, and eating. This is the time to focus your mindful awareness on your pregnancy and your growing baby. It's the perfect time to completely nourish your mind, body, and spirit, knowing that you and your baby will receive direct benefits from this nourishment.

The Necessity of Napping (and Sleeping)

Napping nourishes your body and mind. For some mothers, napping may seem like a luxury or a guilty pleasure, but do not be fooled, napping is actually necessary for rejuvenation for the human body. Researchers at the University of York and Harvard have found that without adequate sleep, your body is prone to memory loss, depression, lack of sex drive, low blood sugar, and reduced energy. Sleep is vital. Our culture has moved away from embracing this necessary and precious act of self-care because we have placed so much value on getting things done. We have detrimentally prioritized the importance of "doing" over "being."

The human body and mind function in cycles of energy called biorhythms. You have high and low energy periods throughout the day. These biorhythms are designed to optimize your body's functions, including tasks like digesting, enhancing your immunity, regenerating your body's cells, and growing your baby. Biorhythms tell your body when to perform certain tasks based on the energy resources it has. The human body is designed to need a nap about eight hours after it wakes up in the morning. For most people this is in the mid-afternoon, between about 2:00 pm to 4:00 pm.

The most rejuvenating type of sleep is the slow wave sleep state of delta. When you achieve this sleep state it allows the memory center in your brain (the hippocampus) to transfer memories to the thinking part of your brain (the neocortex). Slow wave sleeping also allows your brain to reorganize so that it requires less overall energy to function, leaving you with more resources for other activities while awake. However, this sleep state is one that you want to experience at night, not during daytime napping.

For daytime sleep, otherwise known as napping, you want to stay in a lighter sleep state for simple, refreshing rest. Optimal nap times are 15–30 minutes long. The normal sleep cycle is about 90 minutes, and in the first 15–30 minutes the brain is in the alpha state, offering deep relaxation. After the first 30 minutes your mind moves into the delta sleep state, deep sleep. If you nap too long, you can wake up feel sleepy or sluggish.

Pay attention to your body's cues: if you are feeling sleepy, rest. During rest and sleep cycles, the body is able to perform healing activity, release important rejuvenation hormones, and repair itself. Pregnancy places a significant toll on the body and rest is the ultimate medicine.

Rest in the form of napping helps the entire body relax. This allows you to wake up with more creativity, focus, and alertness. If you are not accustomed to napping, you can start by simply paying attention to your body's cues. When your body begins to signal you with signs of sleepiness, (which is simply your body moving into a rest cycle) you might notice some of the following signs:

- Yawning
- Feelings of drowsiness
- Inability to concentrate
- Cravings for caffeine and sugar

It may be common for you to ignore these cues, and perhaps you have used crutches such as caffeine and sugar to enable you to keep going even when your body tells you to rest. Next time you notice these cues, pay attention. For most people, 15–30 minutes is all their body needs to replenish itself. If you are at work, set an alarm for 15–30 minutes later, close your door, and turn off the lights. If you don't have an office, find a safe place to rest. Move into a restful position, put on an eye mask, and focus on moving into your deep belly breathing. If you have a sound machine or an MP3 player, you can play ambient sounds or even purchase music that is specifically designed to get you into a nap state more quickly. Soften your thoughts and relax into the wonderful word of napping. You are sure to wake feeling refreshed.

You deal with stress better when you are well rested, and by now you know that stress management is a critical factor for a healthy pregnancy. If you feel guilty about doing this at work, recognize that nourishing yourself will help keep your body and your pregnancy in a healthier state. It means you are less likely to need to go on bed rest, less likely to have pre-term labor, and from the point of view of your workplace, you will be more efficient and productive after a nap. You can talk to your boss about taking a shorter lunch and using the rest of your lunchtime later in the day for a 15–30 minute nap.

An additional benefit to becoming a prenatal napper is that you will be better at napping after your baby is born. Babies sleep throughout the day and have waking periods at night. If you become accustomed to napping before your baby is born, you will have an easier time napping when your baby naps once she is born. This skill will help you get a full eight hours of sleep over a 24 hour period. Studies show that babies who get plenty of naps sleep better at night. Guess what, mommies do too!

For better nighttime sleep and to increase your slow wave cycles here are some tips from expert sleepers and scientists:

- Warmth and heat help you drift off. Take a warm bath or shower. Cozy up in front of the fireplace. Cuddle up with your partner and discuss the best parts of your day.
- Eat low-to-medium glycemic foods (like whole wheat pasta) shortly before bed. For maximum effect, eat these foods no more than four hours before bed to help encourage slow wave cycles for sleep. A cup of chamomile tea is another great sleep aid. Nuts and seeds are some other good low-glycemic snacks.
- Vigorous exercise in the late afternoon also encourages good nighttime sleep. After work, join your partner or friends for a swim, which is an excellent exercise for pregnancy. Swimming reduces impact on the joints, increases the heart rate, supports the weight of the pregnant body and helps your baby get lined up in the best position for her birth (more to come on that later!). Alternatively, you can take a brisk walk every night after dinner. Walk with your partner or friends; it's a great time to process the events of the day, share your dreams for parenting, and talk about things that really matter!

Sleep is essential and a necessary part of a healthy pregnancy. You can love yourself and your baby by giving yourself permission to enjoy frequent napping and restful sleeping.

A day without a nap is like a cupcake without frosting.
—Terri Guillemets

Stress in the Second Trimester

You have already learned about the importance of deep breathing, yoga, and yawning as great ways to reduce stress, but another way to reduce your stress and enhance your baby's uterine experience is by playing music. Babies respond to music that is played during the second trimester because their hearing is developing and they are learning about their world based on their newly developing senses. Music that has a calming or happy mood has been shown to reduce stress in moms and babies. Babies respond to life-affirming music such as Braham's Lullaby. Interestingly, research shows that babies exposed to music such as rap, heavy metal and even hip hop showed significant signs of stress. Contrary to popular thought, when you play music for your baby, you should not place headphones on your belly. This is partly because it can be too loud for their sensitive developing ears and partly because they should experience music through you. Part of your baby's musical experience is their exposure to the molecules of emotion that your brain is releasing in response to the music. If you play music loud enough for you to hear on your stereo, your baby will be able to hear it as well, with the added benefit that she will experience your feelings relating to the music. Play music you love, music that makes you feel good, music that makes you want to dance.

Eliminating Unsupportive Habits

It is very important to consider what habits you and your partner currently have that need to be changed, limited, or eliminated all together. Since everything you do affects your growing baby, a close examination of you and your partner's routine behaviors is crucial.

Habits that are not supportive to your vitality are often a way to cover up feelings that you wish to suppress. Any action, such as overeating or smoking, that is not in alignment with loving yourself is a separation between you and your source. Identifying unhealthy habits and recognizing the underlying thoughts you have just prior to engaging in these habits is a great first step to begin eliminating them. Often these behaviors are a way of making yourself feel "full," or emotionally satisfied, but this sense of fullness is fleeting and not nourishing. The need for the feeling of fullness is what drives you towards these unhealthy behaviors. Your brain begins to connect the behaviors and the sense of feeling full in ways that make the behaviors habitual. In pregnancy, your habits affect your baby's health, because everything you do during your pregnancy shapes your baby's brain development. As mentioned before, what fires together, wires together.

Breaking habits is difficult, but it can be done. Many studies show that habits in the mother during pregnancy increase the likelihood of the baby developing similar habits as an adult. In fact, studies show that when pregnant mothers eat diets rich in sodium and sugar, their babies tend to grow up with a palate that craves these same foods. You have the power to help your child grow to develop positive and healthy habits.

The key to changing your habits is to first change the thoughts that lead to your unsupportive habits. You must initially recognize that the behavior is not healthy or loving to yourself. Think about the emotion or feeling that is associated with a particular behavior, such as overeating. Does it initially make you feel good? Happy? Joyful? Numb? Next, think about the companion emotion. What do you feel after the behavior is over? Emptiness? Shame? Guilt? Sadness? Disgust? These negative emotions are a sign that you are not loving yourself fully. This ultimately means these habits are not beneficial to your family, your partner, and certainly not to you or your baby.

Take a moment right now. Close your eyes and imagine how you feel after engaging in an unhealthy behavior. Sit for a moment in the companion feeling that arises after the behavior is completed. Now take breath, and imagine participating in a healthy activity that feels good to you, such as taking a walk outside. Connect with the feeling that this healthy behavior brings to you. Now think about which feeling would be more satisfactory as a long-term habit: the resulting emotion of your unhealthy behaviors or the feeling you get when you treat yourself lovingly? Take another breath. Now imagine yourself as a new you, a person who has new and healthier habits. Imagine how your baby feels growing inside a healthier and happier mother. Try to feel gratitude towards yourself, as if you have already made this change in your life. See yourself as already having made these changes in your daily habits, and marinate in this sense of gratitude. You can silently repeat the affirmation, "I am so happy and grateful that I now have _____ as a healthy habit." Repeat this activity daily as you are making your transformation. The next step will be replacing your unhealthy habits with healthy habits.

Common unhealthy or dangerous habits include, but are not limited to:

Obvious unhealthy habits such as:

> Smoking tobacco or marijuana, overuse of caffeine, drinking alcohol, use of illegal or street drugs, habitual and unnecessary use of certain prescription and over-the-counter drugs, any risky behavior, unsafe sex, self abuse or mutilation

Not so obvious unhealthy habits such as:

> Unhealthy diet, overuse of electronics (such as cell phones, computers, video games, and tv), sleep deprivation, relationships with unsupportive or dangerous people, engaging in situations that cause chronic stress, working too much, compulsive spending or shopping, gossiping or participating in conversations that are negative, judgmental, or hurtful

Once you have identified the behavior you wish to change, envision replacement activities that would create a feeling of fullness and contentedness in your life, instead. These should be behaviors that are positive and healthy. What do you do that taps into your creativity and engages your soul and spirit? What do you do that makes you laugh? Do you like to write, cook, read, knit, do yoga or exercise? The options are endless. These are all things that you can begin to direct your energy towards to replace your unhealthy habits. Habits take about thirty days to form. You have about nine months or more to create healthier habits during pregnancy. You can choose to look at your pregnancy as not only the creation of a child and a family, but also the creation of a new you!

It takes time and effort to change habits. You must change your thoughts, your feelings, and your behavior consistently and repetitively to see real change. You need to replace old habits with new experiences. Don't get frustrated if you find yourself occasionally drifting off path. It is normal and to be expected. What is most important is that when you find yourself off your new path, you correct the drift. This requires a renewed, daily commitment to your new path, and a strong resolve to stay the course.

> *And the day came when the risk to remain tight in a bud was more painful than the risk it took to blossom.*
> —Anais Nin

It is always advisable to get professional support and assistance to help address unhealthy or dangerous habits. Talk to your healthcare provider for suggestions and/or see the recommendations in Chapter Two for additional resources.

It is important to be honest with your healthcare provider about your lifestyle. Your doctor or midwife will only be able to recommend the right type of support and/or treatment for you if she knows the whole truth about your lifestyle. The thought of changing habits is not a comfortable one for most people, though some people find that changing unhealthy habits is easier when they know that they will soon become parents.

You may feel a sense of shame or embarrassment associated with some of your unhealthy habits, and that is very normal. These feelings may deter you from openly communicating with your healthcare provider. Keep in mind that your healthcare provider has your best health as her goal and wants to support you in your decision to improve your health. There are many kinds of support available for people who need to make lifestyle changes. Support groups, classes, religious or spiritual support, talk therapy, chiropractic and acupuncture care, nutritional counseling, and, in some cases, prescription medications are all options that can support you during your transition. By being honest with yourself, your partner, and your healthcare provider you are giving your baby the very best version of you.

You're only a thought away from changing your life.
—*Wayne Dyer,* in the movie The Shift

Second Trimester Physical Changes

Please check with your healthcare provider about the safety and efficacy of any treatment for physical challenges in pregnancy.

The good news is that most mothers feel more energetic and comfortable during the second trimester. Though many discomforts from your first trimester have lessened, this period can bring about new physical challenges.

Constipation: Due to the rise in the pregnancy hormone progesterone, your digestive system slows down. This hormone hinders the muscles in the gastrointestinal tract, causing slower digestion. This can cause a host of digestive discomforts like heartburn and constipation. Things you can do to ease discomfort and get things moving include:

- Move your body. This is a prescription for many things that ail the pregnant momma, but it specifically helps with constipation. Walk after meals, practice prenatal yoga, and stretch!
- Increase your intake of water-soluble fiber. This type of fiber can be found in fresh fruits, raw vegetables, and brown rice. Prunes and figs are known for easing constipation.
- Examine your diet. Reduce your consumption of "no value" foods including white flour, sugar, and processed foods.
- Reconsider your prenatal vitamin. As discussed earlier, the type of vitamin you take can impact your body's ability to process foods. Synthetic vitamins often contain high levels

of synthetic iron, which increases the risk of constipation. Consider whole food vitamins.

- Reduce your stress levels. Yes, again it all comes back to stress. Stress keeps things from flowing, literally, in this case!
- Stay hydrated. Drink warm fluids with your meals, not cold drinks. Cold drinks slow down your digestion, while room temperature or warm drinks encourage digestion. Try drinking ginger or fennel tea. Check out your local juice bar or sample some freshly squeezed juice at home. The enzymes in freshly squeezed juices contribute to successful digestion, particularly pineapple, papaya, and mango juices.
- Get a massage. Reflexology and whole body massage can do wonders for the bowels!
- Practice yoga. Many prenatal postures are designed to stimulate the bowels, as a healthy digestive system is considered to be the foundation for a healthy immune system.
- See an acupuncturist who specializes in pregnancy. Acupuncture can be quite helpful for moving chi, releasing energetic blockages, and improving circulation.

Cramps: As your baby begins to grow larger, your uterus increases in size and your ligaments and muscles become stretched. This can cause cramping. This type of cramping is called round ligament pain, which is generally located in the lower abdomen and pelvic area, near the bikini line on the left or right side. This is different from labor contractions or even Braxton Hicks contractions (to be discussed in Part Four). The uterus is surrounded by the round ligaments, which attach to your uterus to hold it in place. During pregnancy they become stretched and elongated and are more prone to spasm if you move quickly or twist and turn your abdomen. This type of cramping can feel tight and sharp and is often relieved by relaxation or a change in position. Most round ligament pain is brief. If you experience cramping or sharp pains in the abdominal area that do not subside quickly, contact your healthcare provider. Things you can do to help prevent round ligament pain and cramping are:

- Avoid twisting or turning your torso quickly. Sleep with pillows supporting your body, as round ligament pain often occurs at night when you roll over quickly in your sleep.
- Practice the yoga posture called Open Legged Child's Pose. To do this, get on your hands and knees and place a pillow on the floor beneath you. Gently push your bottom back towards your heels. Widen your knees and lower your chest towards the pillow beneath you. Soften and rest here.
- Take a warm bath or shower, or use a warm (but not hot) compress on your lower abdomen.
- Stay hydrated.
- Get prenatal massages and chiropractic adjustments to help loosen your muscles and keep your skeletal system aligned.
- Monitor your diet. Lack of salt, magnesium, and calcium can contribute to cramping. Eat calcium and magnesium-rich foods, and salt your food to taste. Great magnesium-rich foods include almonds, cashews, spinach, pumpkin seeds, black beans, and halibut. Calcium rich foods include dark leafy greens, broccoli, cheese, sardines, and yogurt.

You should be concerned and call your healthcare provider if the following are occurring: having waves of contractions (more than four and hour), severe cramping, vaginal bleeding or increased vaginal secretions with cramping, fever, painful urination, or low back pain with cramping. These can be signs of pre-term labor.

Headache: As your estrogen and progesterone levels rise, this can trigger headaches in some women. In addition to hormone changes, there are many reasons you can get a headache during pregnancy, including changes in blood sugar levels and from eating trigger foods like peanuts, aged cheeses, and chocolate. Other common sources of second trimester headaches are stress and fatigue. Listen to your body and if it is "talking" to you with physical discomforts, it is wise to respond. When your body cues you to slow down, heed the warnings. Responding to your body's early cues can help prevent future, more severe discomforts and even pre-term labor. If headaches become a problem, begin to keep a journal to see what you were doing, eating, and what emotions you were feeling just prior to the headache to help identify your common triggers. Some additional ways you can treat the symptoms of headache are:

- Exercise! It's a treatment for so many discomforts in pregnancy. Exercise helps with circulation and also helps to release adrenaline (the stress hormone) from the body, which can contribute to headaches. If traditional exercise does not appeal to you, try a pregnancy movement class such as belly dancing.

- Practice mindful body scan as described earlier in the book. Find a quiet place, lie down, and slowly relax all of your muscles and release tension by focusing on each body part from head to toe. Researchers at Harvard have also found that this type of relaxation has positive benefits for your baby.

- Practice other relaxation techniques. Use three part breathing, deep belly breathing, and diaphragmatic breath in a darkened, quiet room. Try some relaxing yoga postures. These can help with all-over relaxation, as well as improving your posture, which can also be a contributing factor for headaches.

- Get a massage. Massage can help your body release muscle

tension, as well as put you in a deeply relaxed state.

- Stay hydrated and eat small meals often throughout the day to keep your blood sugar levels stable. This helps ensure your body has adequate resources when it needs them.

- Try warm and cold compresses. A warm compress on your eyes and a cold compress on the back of your neck can help alleviate headaches.

- Use a dab of peppermint essential oil on your temples, or on the back of your neck or for inhalation therapy. Some aromatherapy companies make essential oil blends that come in roller ball applications, oil packs, or compresses that are specific for headaches.

- Massage the Ho-Ku point on your hand. This acupressure point can be found in the "v" between the thumb and forefinger. There is usually a bony protrusion on the forefinger at this point that is very sensitive. Massage this area. It is well known for helping to relieve headaches. It is also a great point to massage in labor!

- Try biofeedback. Many chiropractors, doctors, and headache clinics can train you to use this treatment. Biofeedback is a technique to monitor and control your heart rate, blood pressure, and muscle tension. It has been proven to be a very effective headache treatment.

- Chiropractic treatment can help with headaches, both for immediate relief of a headache and also as a preventative measure. Chiropractic manipulation allows the spine to become aligned so that the nerves in the spinal cord can communicate more effectively. It also helps relieve impingements and pressure on spinal nerves.

- Take Acetaminophen. When approved by your healthcare practitioner, this medication is also a common headache treatment. It is not recommended to take Ibuprofen while pregnant. Make certain to follow recommended dosages.

A gentle warning: In the second and third trimester a severe headache can be a sign of preeclampsia, a serious medical condition that requires immediate treatment. If your headaches are accompanied by high blood pressure, blurred or spotty vision, ringing in your ears, nausea, sudden and drastic swelling, pain in upper abdomen, or if your headaches come on very quickly and are very intense, call your healthcare provider right away for quick assessment.

Varicose Veins: This condition can be caused by the increase in the hormone progesterone along with the increase in blood volume during pregnancy. Progesterone relaxes the muscular walls and valves in the veins, which allows for a backflow of blood into the vein. The increasing size and pressure of the uterus can increase the overall pressure in the veins throughout the body. This can lead to varicose veins in the legs, vulva, and rectum (which are called hemorrhoids). Here's what you can do to help prevent varicose veins:

- Avoid standing for long periods at a time. If you have to stand at work, see if you can get a stool to sit on from time to time. On your breaks, find a place to lie down with your feet up for a short while.
- Wear compression hose or socks. This helps keeps pressure on your veins and discourages blood from pooling in the lower extremities.
- Seek out the care of a good prenatal acupuncturist. Acupuncture is a great way to naturally care for varicose veins.
- Eat pineapple. Pineapples contain bromelain that can help reduce the swelling associated with varicose veins. Better yet, make a fruit salsa with pineapple, oranges, apples, and red onions to put on your morning omelet, or to snack on with pita chips. Onions, apples, and citrus fruit contain quercitin, which has anti-inflammatory properties.
- For relief of hemorrhoid discomfort, apply witch hazel

astringent with cotton pads or use hemorrhoid relief products, such as creams and pads, which can be found at any pharmacy. Stay hydrated and eat a diet high in soluble fiber.

Carpal Tunnel Syndrome: Between the wrist bones and wrist ligament runs a canal called the carpal tunnel. Inside this canal is the median nerve, which gives sensation to the index, middle, ring finger, and thumb. During pregnancy, the increase in fluid retention can put pressure on the median nerve, leading to the symptoms of carpal tunnel syndrome. These include numbness, pins and needles sensation, and aching and tingling in the wrist and fingers. If you are experiencing these symptoms, please consult with a healthcare provider. This condition, if related to fluid retention in pregnancy, generally resolves after the birth. Some natural ways to deal with the symptoms are:

- Be aware of how you sleep. Try to not bend your affected wrist or sleep on it. Before you go to bed and when you wake up, roll your wrists and wiggle out your fingers.
- Make sure your workstation is ergonomic. This means that it is designed to put the least amount of stress on your body. Your computer monitor should be placed so that you can look straight at it. Your keyboard should be placed so that your hands, wrist, and fingers are in one plane, not bent during use. Your wrist should not have to rest on the sharp edge of a desk.
- Use ice wisely. Short applications of an ice pack on the wrist for 5–15 minutes a day can help reduce swelling.
- Get acupuncture, acupressure, or chiropractic adjustments. These treatments increase blood flow and reduce swelling to the carpal tunnel.
- Verify you are getting enough B6 (1.9 mg per day) from natural food sources, including potatoes, chicken, salmon, pork, chick peas, bananas, and mangoes.

- Try prenatal yoga. There are many yoga positions that help increase flexibility in your wrists, as well as reduce congestion, and improve blood flow.
- If your symptoms persist, your healthcare provider may recommend wearing a wrist brace or physical therapy.

Sciatic Pain: It is very common to experience irritation of the sciatic nerve during pregnancy, which results in sciatic nerve pain. The sciatic nerve runs from the low back, across the buttocks, down the legs, and into the feet. Sciatic nerve pain can be caused by uterine compression or your baby's position, tension in the abdominal muscles, postural changes, poor posture, spinal compression, or rarely, spinal disc damage. Some ways to deal with sciatic nerve pain:

- Use pelvic rocking. Get on your hands and knees and rock your pelvis back and forth and in circles. You can practice open-legged child's pose, as well.
- Use hydrotherapy. Take a warm bath, shower, or use a warm pack on the area causing pain.
- Get a massage. Often massage therapists will focus on relaxing and releasing the psoas and gluteal muscles, which are often triggers for sciatic pain.
- Sit on an exercise or birth ball and practice pelvic rocking. Wiggle your hips, and make pelvic circles, which help to relax your lower back.
- Practice prenatal yoga. Many of the hands and knees positions in yoga can help with sciatic pain. Be sure to tell your instructor that you are having sciatic pain so that she can offer you alternative positioning that won't aggravate the condition.
- Get good chiropractic care and/or physical therapy. Often sciatic nerve pain can be relieved with these treatments.

Pregnancy discomforts are normal. They are usually signs that your body is working according to design. While it is important to talk openly and honestly with your healthcare provider about concerns that you may have, be aware that too many calls to your healthcare providers office about normal pregnancy discomforts may lead to unnecessary medical interventions. Most discomforts can be treated naturally, without medical intervention. Use conscious agreement when dealing with physical discomforts. If you sense that you should call your healthcare provider, call her!

While your second trimester does have its discomforts, it's often the perfect time to take advantage of the energy and vitality you feel now. This is great time to plan weekend getaways with your partner or friends, shop for the nursery, participate in pregnancy exercise classes, and simply enjoy this time.

Part Three

Activities for Nourishing

Meditations

This section includes a couple of meditations that your partner or friend can read to you or that you can read to yourself. You can also record yourself reading these meditations to practice anytime, including during your labor. If you chose to read to yourself, close your eyes and let your mind take you where it may after you have read a particular meditation.

The Four Elements Meditation

Sit in a mindful presence. Breathing in, feel the movement of air bring you into a place of stillness. Follow your breath as it moves in and out, allowing your attention to rest on the ebb and flow of the breath. As you become more and more present, honoring yourself in this space of awareness, meet yourself in this space with gratefulness for the elements around you: wind, water, earth, and fire. You can draw on these elements to create a peace and mindfulness within yourself.

Wind: As you breathe in, allow your focus to rest on the element of wind. This element has an energy and force within its movement. Wind is the source of our breath, feel its power moving through your body. As your inhalation moves through you, feel it expanding the back of the throat, the lungs, the diaphragm, and abdomen. Feel the expansion in your pelvis. Know that as you invite the wind to move within your body, you open up to its inspiration. As you move through your next exhalation, feel the contraction of the abdomen, diaphragm, and lungs. Release tension, carbon dioxide, and any emotions that don't serve you. Allow them to flow out on your breath, mingling with the wind and moving away from you as your body prepares to inhale another sip of pure and powerful wind. There is no such thing as a block or an obstacle to wind. The wind simply moves around it, finds a new pathway, embraces and caresses that which at first seemed to be an obstacle. Remember the wind in pregnancy and in labor if at any time you feel you need to move around or through something. Allow its power and presence to saturate your breath and create a sense of fluidity. Use the power of the wind now. If there is something within you that you have been feeling a resistance to or wish to release, allow the energy of wind to help you move through it. Imagine a symbol, a word, or a thought to represent this issue or challenge and see it begin to float before you. As it becomes more present for you, imagine that your breath is actually moving in and out through this symbol. As your breath moves in and out and flows around this object, see it beginning to dissipate, to dissolve and float in tiny specks out and away from you to be returned to the wind. Continue to breathe as you allow this vision to slowly fade and return to focus only on the inhalation and exhalation moving through your body. As you meditate on wind, remember that in the future as the wind blows, it is a reminder to breathe, to be inspired.

Water: Shift your focus to the element of water. The element of water nourishes you, hydrates your body, quenches your thirst, and allows you to float, swim, and relax. In fact, the water in the ocean has a similar makeup to the amniotic fluid surrounding your baby. This water cradles your baby, allowing her to dip and dive and turn to find her most comfortable resting place, head down and facing your spine. Water is the element that regenerates your body. It flushes contaminates and toxins through your system and releases unwanted impurities from your body. Water is necessary to every cell in your body and to your baby's body. It is the basic building block of humanity. Water helps absorb your pain as you float and soak in a bath. Water gets expelled from your body through sweat and tears when you need to release toxins or emotions from the body. Water is your great protector and benefactor. Just like wind, water too can move around objects. Instead of being blocked by things that seem immovable, water will simply mold to whatever container it is placed in, or will move around objects trying to block its path. You can be like water, adapt to your environment, and be happy where you are. Water can also create channels and wear rough surfaces smooth. Focus on this amazing element; imagine your body swaying back and forth, from side to side as though waves from the ocean are gently caressing your body. Feel the power of water and its protective energy. As you gently sway back and forth, connect to what the element of water can bring to you. Slowly return and focus simply on inhaling and exhaling and the movement of your breath. Bring your body back to stillness. Use the meditation of water during your pregnancy and labor if you feel blocked.

'Fire: Bring your focus to the element of fire. Fire is the element that brings energy and heat to your world. It also allows for regeneration and starting anew. Fire symbolizes passion and strength. Fire connects you with the sun and stars. Fire warms your planet with its sunlight. Fire can light your way when you are in the darkness. Fire is the element associated with passion, creativity, and desire. It is the element you can draw on during your pregnancy and birth when you need additional strength and when you need renewal. As you meditate on this element, if there is an issue that you need to shine light on, or an area of your life in which you wish to start fresh, allow that idea to come before you now. Imagine a symbol, word, or thought to symbolize that issue or topic. Let that image float before you, becoming clearer with each inhalation. Imagine that at your heart's center, a warm fire begins to glow. It is a protective flame that generates only warmth and protection. Allow that flame to become infused with any color that feels safe and protective for you. With each inhalation visualize the fire growing, and with each exhalation see it spreading light on the symbol before you. Allow the light from your own fire to illuminate and bring clarity to this issue for you. (Allow for quiet meditation here for about two minutes.) Begin to return to your breath, focusing only on the movement of the breath through your body, moving back into stillness. Know that any time in your pregnancy or birth you can draw on the element of fire to offer you protection and illumination.

Earth: We now bring our attention to the element of earth. From fiery lava, the earth is transformed. The water on the earth, from oceans to rivers, mold and transform the earth's appearance. The wind moves over and around the earth, helping to support life on the earth. As the three elements work together, earth becomes a life-giving space that nourishes, protects, and generates. Staying connected with the earth allows you to stay connected to all elements at the same time, creating a sense of balance deep within yourself. As you breathe, feel your connection to the earth growing and deepening. Imagine you are a tree sprouted from the earth and your feet become roots and keep you firmly connected to the earth beneath you. As you allow your breath to flow through your body, feel your connection to all the elements surrounding you. Feel the wind moving through your body, feel the flow of water gently washing around you, feel the heat and light of the sun shining on you, feel the earth pressed against your feet. You are now connected to all of the elements, and thus are whole. Feel the sense of safety in the elements and the power they have to transform your pregnancy and birth. Know that at any moment in time you can draw on this image to bring balance and connection to your spirit.

Stay in this meditation for a few moments.

Bring your focus back to your breathing. Slow your inhalation and exhalation. Feel your mind retuning back to your body and feel your breathing return to normal. Open your eyes, feeling refreshed and peaceful.

Intention Setting

This meditation is designed to help you to listen in to your inner voice. During meditation you can become aware of what your mind, body and spirit really need. When you become aware of your needs, you can set intentions to help you meet those needs. Intentions are plans that help you move towards your higher purpose. This meditation is designed to be practiced while in a sitting position.

Allow your eyelids to close and your eyes to relax. Release any tension between your brows. Tune in to your breathing. For the next few moments, simply allow yourself to listen to your breath. Don't try to change or manipulate your breathing. Simply become a non-judgmental observer of your breath. Notice how your breath flows through your body. Does your chest expand? Your belly? Is the inhalation or exhalation longer? Is there a pause between breaths or does your breath loop into one continuous circle? Is there a place in your body where the breath seems to catch and pause, or does your breath flow evenly throughout your body?

Now that you have observed your breath, purposefully slow down your breathing. Intentionally inhale, bringing the breath into the body like delicious sips of air, filling a vessel. Fill the vessel of your body from lung to diaphragm to abdomen. Allow for a short pause between inhalation and exhalation. Exhale slowly, feel the air pour out of your body, releasing, softening, letting go. Continue breathing in this manner for the next few breaths until you can let go of your thinking mind and simply allow the deep breath to move through the body without having to think about it.

Begin to slowly bring your focus on the space between your brows, sometimes called the third eye. This space actually houses a fascinating gland called the pineal gland that is stimulated in times of deep meditation. This gland releases hormones that help alter your mental state into an alpha or relaxed state where your subconscious and conscious mind can meet. When this gland is stimulated, it cues your body into a deep sense of well-being and creativity.

Bring your attention to this space between your brows. You may, in fact, wish to imagine that your breath is beginning to flow in and out through this space. As your breath moves through this space, it creates an opening for energy movement. Feel this space warming and energizing. Spend the next few moments simply focusing on this space and breathing in the manner that feels best to you.

Now that you have stimulated your pineal gland, your body and mind are ready for intention setting. As you breathe deeply, invite an intention to present itself to you. Do not force an intention to come to you, simply invite an intention to manifest itself within your thoughts. Try not to judge the intention, and simply allow whatever your spirit needs to present itself to you. It may seem odd or strange to you, but know that in this state of mindfulness, the subconscious is speaking to you.

Once the intention is clear, feel your breath moving in and out through this thought. Invite the intention to manifest itself in your life. Imagine this intention becoming a part of your life, so that it becomes a part of you. Feel gratitude for this intention being a part of your life.

Return to your breath. Inhaling and exhaling, feeling relaxed and peaceful. As you allow your breath pattern to normalize, feel good about the intention you have set.

Part Three:
Keynotes for Nourishing

Your baby's emotional center of her brain develops during the second trimester, so creating peace and love in your life is critical now. Try incorporating Fetal Love Breaks throughout the day to send your baby a dose of love hormones.

Nourishing your partner relationship has never been more important because your child starts to have a relationship with her father well before she is born by sharing your emotions and feelings.

Make time to talk with your partner about his concerns, worries, and fears. Make a plan as a family to address these issues before the baby arrives.

Practicing conscious agreement in your partner relationship means being aware of your ability to positively communicate. Remember to practice H.A.L.T, don't engage in important conversations when hungry, angry, lonely, or tired.

Practice responsibility in your words and actions.

Stay in the present moment.

Observe yourself in communication.

Develop your listening skills.

⚷ Nap, nap, nap and get at least six hours of sleep a night. Nap at least 15–30 minutes during the day. For better nighttime sleep, use warmth and heat, eat low-to-medium glycemic foods within four hours of going to sleep, and exercise in the late afternoon.

⚷ Focus on eliminating or reducing unhealthy habits.

Part Four

The Third Trimester of Pregnancy

B-O-N-**D**

D stands for Deciding

"Stay committed to your decisions, but stay flexible in your approach."
—**Tony Robbins**

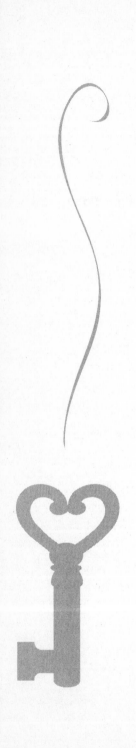

Chapter Fourteen
Decisions During Pregnancy

*"You are constructing your own reality with the choices you make...
or don't make. If you really want a healthy pregnancy and joyful
birth, and you truly understand that you are the one in control, then
you must examine what you have or haven't done so far to create
the outcome you want."*
—Kim Wildner, Mother's Intention: How Belief Shapes Birth

The third trimester is a time when you naturally move from imagination into reality. All of the dreams you have had are about to manifest into your new family. This is the time to make some concrete decisions about where you want to have your baby, what you want your labor and birth to be like, and how you want to practice early parenting in the first months of being a new mom. It is normal to feel consumed by thoughts about preparing for your baby's arrival.

Nesting is a primal instinct that most mothers experience as they prepare to welcome their babies. In the third trimester, you to begin to withdraw from the business of the external world and start to prepare your nest. The decisions you make now can lay a strong foundation for a gentler, calmer postpartum experience for you and your baby. As you make plans to welcome your newborn, your baby is getting ready for her exciting journey into a new world. Your baby begins establishing memory, experiencing rapid brain growth, and learning at astounding rates to help her transition to a new life in your arms. Your baby is highly tuned in to your world.

Your baby begins to determine if the world is a place of security or one of danger by reacting to stimuli from the world outside. Your attention to your baby's needs prepare her to greet her new world with trust, calmness, and a sense of security.

What's Up, Baby?

Weeks 28–32: Your little one weighs approximately 3.5 pounds and will be about 16.5 inches long. She is sleeping and waking according to her own rhythms and cycles, regulating herself as her body continues to grow. She is experiencing rapid eye movement sleep, otherwise known as REM, which means she dreams while she sleeps. She already has a rich emotional life and her brain is rapidly connecting billions of neurons, shaping her idea of the world outside the womb. Her heart rate will respond by slowing down when you talk directly to her in a calming demeanor. She is deeply connected to your voice. Her milk teeth have developed below her gum line. Her eyes are capable of moving in their sockets and she can follow the light from a flashlight shined on your belly. In fact, her eyes can even detect the differences between sunlight and artificial light, and her pupils dilate in response to changes in light. Her taste buds are maturing, and she can respond to flavors in the amniotic fluid by either gulping or grimacing. Your diet is influencing her palate, and eating a nutritious diet rich in flavor now can help your baby develop healthy eating patterns later on. Her lungs have developed to the point that she would have a great chance of survival even if she were born right now. The hair on her head is becoming thicker, as are her eyebrows and eyelashes. Her body is becoming more and more capable of functioning independently. Her bone marrow begins producing red blood cells, which transport nutrients and eliminate waste throughout her body. Her body is also beginning to store minerals like iron, phosphorus, and calcium, which will help her grow efficiently as a newborn. Your baby also begins to explore her own body by touching her toes, feeling her arms and hands, and grasping at her umbilical cord. This helps her become familiar with the sensation of touch. Her digestive tract is maturing, preparing for her first nourishing meals of colostrum (the newborn milk your breasts make). Towards the end of this period, her body will focus on creating fat stores and increasing the muscle mass in her tiny body.

Weeks 32–36: Your baby is growing rapidly now, which means she is much more snug inside the uterus. You'll feel her movements intensely now, as there is not as much space for her to wiggle about. She has grown to approximately 5.5 pounds and can be up to 18.5 inches long. Your baby's genitalia are maturing, if you have a boy his testicles will begin their descent into the scrotum, and if you are having a girl her clitoris is increasing in size. Your calcium intake will have a direct effect on the development of your baby's bones and teeth, so choose healthy sources of calcium for your diet, like dark greens, hard cheeses, and fish with edible bones, such as sardines. Your baby is learning how to digest by drinking amniotic fluid and urinating throughout the day. She begins to lay down fat stores in her body and gains about half a pound every week. Her body is beginning to regulate its own temperature. However, if she were born now she would still need to be kept in constant skin-to-skin contact with you or stay in an incubator to keep her warm. She will open her eyes when she is awake and close her eyes when sleeping. Her immune system is being boosted by antibodies to prepare her for a new environment once she is born.

Weeks 36–42: Much of your baby's mature brain growth occurs in the last four weeks of pregnancy. This process allows her to breastfeed better, maintain her temperature, and interact with her environment. During these final weeks, babies often begin to make their way down into the pelvis head first, which is called lightening or dropping. Ideally, your baby will be positioned so that her back is rested against your belly and she is facing your backside. This is known as the anterior position and it makes her journey down the birth canal easier when her birthday arrives. The fine hair that covered your baby's body, lanugo, is now disappearing and her skin is becoming smooth. Additionally, the white coating called vernix, that protects your baby's skin from the watery environment, is diminishing. She begins to store her first bowel movements, meconium, in her intestines. Her body has grown and prepared her for her destiny, to be your child. She is ready to be welcomed into your arms.

What's Up, Mama?

Are we there yet? You may find yourself increasingly tired of being pregnant and wishing that your estimated due date had already arrived. Your weight will increase at a rate of about a pound a week, due to the rapid growth of your baby. You may be increasingly uncomfortable as your baby grows larger and takes up even more room. Braxton Hicks contractions are a normal part of this last trimester. Braxton Hicks are warm-up contractions that prepare your uterus for the real deal: labor. You may feel hot flashes as the hormone estrogen fluctuates, making night sweats a common event. Back pain and joint pain are also normal during the third trimester. You may experience more growth and tenderness in your breasts and some milk leakage is normal. Leg cramps can occur, and are more often experienced during the nighttime hours. As the uterus stretches and your baby grows even larger it is more common to experience round ligament pain. Your belly button may become an outie, but don't worry, it will go back to normal after delivery. This is actually a sign that your baby is lined up for labor. Your hands and feet may be slightly swollen now, due to the increased pressure from your uterus. Additionally, the hormone progesterone causes the kidneys to retain more sodium during pregnancy, which can cause swelling. Once your baby moves down into the pelvis you may find it easier to breathe and mealtime may be more pleasurable, but you will feel more pelvic pressure. Your baby's descent causes even more pressure on the bladder, which leads to more frequent urination. You might begin to "waddle" due to the increased pressure of baby's body resting in your pelvis. Your duck-like swagger is a sign your baby will soon be in your arms. Towards the end of the third trimester, your cervix may start to open and the protective plug inside may discharge. This is called the release of the mucous plug. It is also common to see some slight spotting, which is due to the stretching of the cervix. (If this happens before 37 weeks call your caregiver.) Your estimated due date is approaching and your body is preparing for baby's arrival without you even needing to think about it. There is an increase in the hormone relaxin, which helps the ligaments attached to the pelvis become more flexible for birth. This can cause you to feel clumsier, as your ligaments stretch. Try not to overdo it, and get plenty of rest and fluids. Remember your due date is just an estimate, and only a very small percentage of women spontaneously go into labor on or before their due date. Get ready to meet the love of your life!

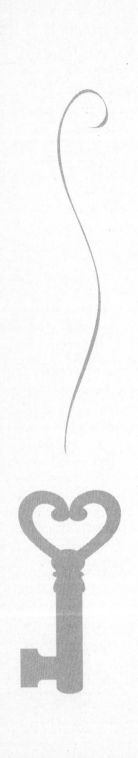

Chapter Fifteen

Keys to Slowing Down and Nesting

"Take rest. A field that has rested gives bountiful crop."
—Ovid

Slowing down is key to easing into your third trimester. As the hormones of nesting begin to take hold, you will find yourself in a state of reorganization and planning. It's easy to become overwhelmed with endless to-do lists and forget about the most essential preparation of all—slowing down and tuning in to the motherbaby bond.

Many cultures around the world honor this period in pregnancy and encourage the motherbaby bond. Traditional Japanese families believe that babies are influenced by the mother's thoughts, as well as by music. Pregnant Japanese women are encouraged to look at beautiful images, think positive thoughts, and listen to calming, beautiful music. In China, pregnant women are encouraged to avoid being critical of others, as it is believed any criticism will cause the pregnant mother's baby to take on these traits. Pregnancy is viewed as a time when a woman has happiness in her body. In Hawaiian tradition, babies are raised in the spirit of Ohana, or family bond. Babies and children are called keiki, meaning seedling. Hawaiians wish to grow their children from the nourishing source of love.

A wonderful way to honor this time of nesting and preparation is to have a blessingway performed for you. A blessingway is a very different celebration than a baby shower, though sometimes the two are combined. This ceremony originates from the Native American Navajo practices to honor and bless the transition to motherhood.

The actual Navajo word for blessingway is Hozho which has multiple meanings and encompasses all things good, beautiful, and in harmony. The blessingway ceremony honors the sacred rite of passage that a mother is going through. It can be a profound experience for all involved and typically is a ceremony where only women are present.

The first step to the blessingway ritual is to organize a gathering of those who support and love you unconditionally. Often the ceremony begins with singing or storytelling and a lighting of candles. The first person lights a candle and says, for example, "I am Laurel, daughter of Jane, granddaughter of Louise, and mother of Trevor and Ryan." The next person lights a candle and shares their family story until the circle ends at the mother to be. Everyone uses their own candle to light one large candle in the center of the circle as the pregnant mother shares her story. These same candles can be lit again as a vigil during the mother's labor. Next, the guests share something intimate with the group about their feelings for the mother and baby and their wishes for her future. Small and sacred gifts are given to the mother at this time. These gifts are typically handmade or of personal significance.

Next, the mother is given a footbath. Her feet are rubbed with blue cornmeal for purification, and then soaked in a warm bowl of water that may contain essential oils and flower petals. During the footbath, she is given a hand and head massage. After the footbath, there is time for storytelling. Personal and positive stories of courage regarding parenting, birth, and being a woman or mother are told. Sometimes a mother has her belly cast at this point, or has a henna painting done on her belly. Belly casting involves making a plaster mold of the belly and torso, which can be kept as a keepsake of the pregnancy. Henna art is an Indian tradition where the vegetable dye henna is painted in intricate patterns and symbols on the skin to celebrate a rite of passage. Finally, the ceremony ends with sharing delicious homemade foods. Some additional activities used at blessingways are:

- Bead ceremony: the guests bring a bead that symbolizes something they want to convey to the mother. The bead is given to the mother and a necklace is strung for her to wear during her labor as a reminder of her blessings.
- Mother's wish book: guests have an opportunity to write something personal for the new mother, as well as offer wishes for her journey into motherhood.
- String ceremony: a skein of yarn is placed in the center of the circle and a prayer or poem is read. The yarn is then looped around the mother's wrist and subsequently wrapped around the wrists of all of the guests. This symbolizes a deep connection between the mother and all of the women present. The string is then cut and small sections are tied around each woman's wrist. The bracelets are worn until the baby is born.

The blessingway is a time when you can feel completely honored, loved, and celebrated. Many women are choosing to have blessingways instead of or as a part of a traditional baby shower. The focus is on you, the mother, and the celebration is a heartwarming way to step into motherhood.

In addition to the celebrations that may occur during the nesting period, the third trimester is the time to begin making plans for the arrival of your baby. Having the intimate and important discussions that matter to the long-term health of your family is an important part of nesting. It may sound confusing to think about slowing down and nesting at the same time, but this is the way of motherhood. As you take the time to focus on the motherbaby bond, you can tap into your inner wisdom. This will help you make important decisions, such as those discussed later in this chapter.

As you begin nesting, you might conjure up ideas about whom you think your child will be one day, how she will laugh, what she will do when she grows up. What are you contributing to this unique little person inside of you? Remember that your emotions help develop the emotional center in your baby's brain, the amygdala, and determine how she balances her emotions. When mothers learn that their emotions help develop their baby's personality, it is common for them to begin to worry about times they have been stressed or angry during their pregnancy. Remind yourself instead to focus on your blessings at this time. Be in a state of gratitude as often as you can. Try to move from a state of mind of "it's hopeless" to "I am hopeful." Sit for a moment and begin to count your blessings. Focus on the many things that you have gratitude for in this moment. Having an attitude of gratitude can help keep you in a state of positive emotion.

Try this activity:

Find a beautiful basket, bowl, or box that you can symbolize as the nest you are creating for your child. Reflect on all of the gifts you wish to give your child. Some examples might be security, love, happiness, and sense of family. Find an item that represents each of these gifts; for example, a stone in the shape of a heart to symbolize love. Place these items in your nest. Make note that most of the time, the things you really want for your child do not cost money, but instead involve time spent with your child. Next, write a letter to your child sharing the meaning behind these gifts you want to give to your child and take a picture of your nest. This can be a wonderful keepsake. You may wish to share this activity with your partner. Once your symbolic nest is completed, spend a few days reflecting on the actual nest you are creating for your baby. What does your real nest look like? Does your home and life reflect the qualities that you admire? What, if anything, do you need to change? Remember that pregnancy is an opportunity, a gift that you are given to create the nest of your choice for your new family.

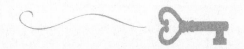

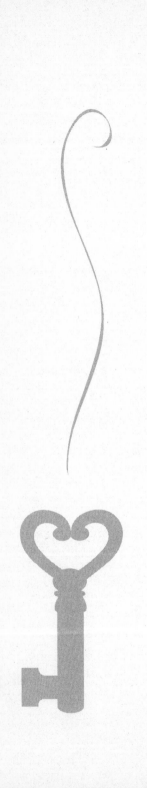

Chapter Sixteen

Important Discussions and Considerations

"Whatever you are, whatever you do, your baby will get it. Anything you eat, any worries that are on your mind will be for him or her. Can you tell me that you cannot smile? Think of the baby, and smile for him, for her, for the future generations."
—**Thich Nhat Hanh, Being Peace**

Your mind begins to run in circles in the third trimester. The people in your life love you and want the best for you. They offer opinions about your choices, which can confuse you. You may find yourself awake all night considering all of your parenting and birthing options. In this section, some of these important decisions will be discussed. Remember to keep conscious agreement at the center of your decision-making process.

Before you move into the decision-making process, it can be helpful to create a birthing vision board. A vision board is a visual representation of your aspirations. It is used as a tool to help you shed light on the things that matter the most to you as a mother and clarify what is it that you really want during the birthing process. It is an activity that helps you to place your *attention* on your *intention*. In a way, vision boards are like a prayer, they can connect you to your source and illuminate your dreams, hopes, and wishes.

Using the keys to conscious agreement, you (and your partner) can create your unique vision board to represent the birth that you dream of. This may seem like a strange or new age thing to do, but it is actually a way to help your brain identify your heart's desires so they can be realized. A vision board can be your map towards a great birth experience. Think of how a successful business starts. It begins with a business plan that maps out a mission and vision and how the business will get there. A birth vision board is a great replacement for a traditional birth plan.

The part of your brain that is at work during your birth is your mammalian brain. This part of your brain controls the hormones that help your labor and birth unfold. This part of your brain is much more visual than verbal, so choose images and colors that visually soothe you. You should choose words and images that make you feel good and portray your thoughts about your baby and your birth. For example, you might choose an image of a beach if that represents a feeling of peace for you. A vision board can in fact be a type of meditation or prayer.

Remember conscious agreement for your birth vision board:

Step One: Separate yourself from external influences. Go to a quiet place where you can be uninterrupted. Bring poster board or a large sheet of paper, markers or crayons, magazines you love, pictures, scissors, glue, and anything else you might want to decorate your board with.

Step Two: Get quiet and pause. Start by quieting your mind and beginning either meditation or prayer. Visualize yourself as a mother. Visualize your baby. What does that bond look and feel like to you? How do you want this to be expressed in your labor and delivery? Try not to force ideas, just open up. As your intentions come to you, breathe them in. Feel them becoming a part of you with each breath. Stay in this quiet space for as long it feels comfortable to you.

Step Three: Listen In. This time "listening" involves paying attention to the visual images in the magazines surrounding you. Begin by selecting images that seem to resonate with your intentions. Next arrange them on the paper into a shape or flow that appeals to you. Place a picture of yourself in the center of your vision board so that the images surround you, and you are the center of all of these intentions. There may be areas on your vision board that you have not filled up, white space. This is okay. Leave yourself some space to be open to ideas that may still come to you.

Step Four: Decide and commit. Once you have created your birth vision board, hang it up. Put it in a place where it is visible not only to yourself but also to those who are important to you. Use it as a tool to discuss your hopes and your plans. Share it with your doctor or midwife. Show it to your doula. Bring it to your birth. It's a piece of art that expresses your birth intentions.

You may wish to create a vision board surrounding anything in your life, including your baby, your marriage, your parenting style, or your family. Save your vision boards; they will become unique historical journals of who you were when you created them. It is always fascinating to look back and see what your intentions were and how they manifested in your life. This is a great way to teach your children to tune into their hearts' desires, as well.

A note from Tracy and Laurel: Even if it seems a little strange, we whole-heartedly encourage you to try creating a vision board. Do it with an open heart and mind, and you will be surprised to look back and see how your prayers were answered.

Now that you have considered your wishes for your birth with the vision board, you will need to take a closer look at some of the options you will have during your labor and delivery. It's time to make some decisions. Keep in mind that these decisions are deeply personal and should be based on how you and your partner feel, not the opinions of others. While having discussions with important people in your life might help you discover your innermost feelings, be careful to not be overly influenced by other people's opinions if they do not reflect your own. Before any final decision is made, go back to conscious agreement, which can help you tune in to how *you* feel.

The reality is that your pregnancy will last approximately nine full months, and parenting will last a lifetime. This may make the decisions concerning a typical 24 hour labor seems comparatively less significant, however your birth experience impacts you and your baby physically, emotionally, and spiritually. It is likely that you will remember your birth experience for the rest of your life. Therefore, thoughtful consideration of your options is a wise investment for your family.

Perceptions of Pain

> *"We have a secret in our culture...and it's not that birth is painful. It's that women are strong."*
> —Laura Stavoe Harm

If you are like most women, you have already spent some time thinking about how you will handle the pain of labor and birth. It is completely normal to have some fear about this. Any time you are faced with the unknown, it is common to move into a fear response. The following information can help you reframe the way you think about pain in labor.

The pain that you feel in labor is different from any other type of pain you experience in your life. It is actually a sign that your body is working for you, not a sign of illness or injury. The physical causes of labor pain include the movement of the baby, stretching of your ligaments, opening or dilation of your cervix, pressure of your baby moving through the birth canal, and uterine muscle fatigue.

However, emotional factors can affect the perception of pain as well. These include, but are not limited to, anxiety (which increases bodily tension), fear, lack of support, previous experiences with pain, beliefs about your body and your ability to birth, and unexpected occurrences, such as medical interventions. Your environment also affects how you feel and deal with pain. When you have the freedom to move around, use the comfort techniques of your choice, and have access to nourishment and hydration, you will find that your perception of pain is decreased.

Believe it or not, your mind has already formed an opinion about birth based on subconscious programming. What you believe is based on the culture you grew up in and the media that you have been exposed to. Your belief systems regarding your body and birthing have a lot to do with how you will perceive pain during your labor. Close your eyes for a moment and visualize a woman in labor. Think about where she is and what she is doing. What comes to mind? Where did you get that image? Is this the way you WANT to give birth, or is it simply the way you think most women actually have a baby? The most common modern image of a woman laboring is one of her lying on her back and in terrible pain. This image is perpetuated by the media, our society, and some healthcare professionals, who have likely not witnessed birth without medical management. It is not an accurate portrayal of the normal process of labor and birth. You are not the victim of your contractions. Your labor is not meant to punish you. When you are in an environment of safety and security (your nest), your body is designed to help you cope with the sensations of labor and birth. Contractions are your body's way of bringing your baby into the world. Your body is working for you, not against you.

===

MYTH: Labor pain is continuous.

REALITY: Contractions are intermittent with rest in between. In a typical 24-hour labor, only 3 hours is actual contraction time. The majority of your labor is downtime.

MYTH: Pain is unmanageable without medication.

REALITY: There are many natural techniques and comfort measures that have been shown to decrease pain perceptions, improve relaxation, and shorten labor.

MYTH: Labor is intense and fast from the very beginning.

REALITY: Labor usually starts slowly and gradually intensifies. Your body has a chance to adjust and release comfort hormones to help with the pain.

MYTH: Because women tend to vocalize or moan in labor it means they are in great pain.

REALITY: Vocalization and moaning is a natural response during labor. It helps decrease the sensation of pain and softens the birth passage for the baby by relaxing the perineal muscles.

MYTH: Pain is a sign that something is wrong.

REALITY: Sensation in labor is actually a sign that your body is working effectively.

===

Dana's Story

Like many women, Dana had not planned on getting pregnant. However, as her estimated due date draws near, she becomes more excited about being a mother. Dana is single and lives with her mom, Anita. Dana has had a long day at work. Being on her feet all day is exhausting and she is happy to finally be home. She grabs the remote and is pleased to find her favorite guilty pleasure on T.V., a popular series about hospital birth. Even though Dana knows that this show increases her anxiety about her upcoming birth (she plans on a natural delivery), she feels strangely attracted to it. On this episode, the pregnant woman is out of control, yelling at her husband and screaming for an epidural. This scene reminds Dana of a conversation she recently had with her best friend who was sharing about her own birth experience. Dana begins to notice that her stomach is hurting, her palms are sweaty, and she feels uneasy. (Is Dana in conscious agreement?)

The show ends and Dana realizes she does not even want to eat dinner. Her mother, Anita, arrives home just as Dana is turning off the television. She tells her mother she is not feeling well and heads off to bed early. Several hours later she wakes up having contractions. Dana calls for her mother. Despite what they learned in childbirth classes, Anita is not comfortable with her daughter laboring at home "where anything can go wrong." They head to the hospital right away.

Upon their arrival, Dana has a cervical check and is found to be three centimeters dilated. Even though she is in only in early labor, the hospital admits her anyway. The nurse has Dana get in bed, starts an I.V., and monitors the baby. A few hours go by, and although Anita has tried to keep her daughter comfortable, Dana is in a lot of pain and seems be losing it. She tells her mom she wants an epidural, leaving all plans of her natural childbirth behind. All she can think about is the scary birth she watched on T.V. earlier.

At shift change, a new nurse, Henrietta, steps in to meet Dana and her mom. Henrietta asks Dana how she is doing and Dana immediately says, "I want my epidural." Henrietta glances at the chart and comments, "It says here you want to go natural. Why the change in plans?" Dana bursts into tears, sobbing, "I am so afraid." Henrietta pulls up a chair, holds Dana's hand and softly says, "Talk to me."

Between contractions, Dana shares her fears about everything she has seen on T.V. and questions her ability to manage the pain on her own. Henrietta replies, "Well, you have to work with your body. Let's get you out of bed and change things up. Then we can see if you still want an epidural." As Henrietta helps get Dana onto a birthing ball, she shows Anita how and where to massage Dana's back to help with the pain. Dana starts to move around on the ball and Henrietta tells her about the women in her family back in Jamaica. She shares that they believe birth is a gift and that movement and singing help to bring babies into their mother's arms. Dana feels instantly soothed when she hears Henrietta humming softly.

Anita can tell that the atmosphere has changed and her daughter seems more relaxed. Dana closes her eyes, hums, and visualizes her baby's face. As she starts to relax, she begins using the deep breathing techniques she learned in childbirth class. An epidural is no longer on Dana's mind and she is working with each contraction as it comes. She has made a shift from fear to confidence with the guidance and support from Henrietta and her mother. How did Dana's belief systems contribute to her perception of pain? What helped her make a shift?

Location, Location, Location

Pregnant women are encouraged to be as active as possible because of the wide array of benefits that exercise and movement offer. One additional benefit is that movement can help get your baby lined up in the best possible position for your labor and birth. Optimal fetal positioning is a technique that was originally developed by midwife Jean Sutton and childbirth educator Pauline Scott. They discovered that maternal movement and positioning affects the way a baby positions herself in the pelvis and can improve the outcome of labor.

Toward the end of your pregnancy, your baby takes cues from nature and starts to settle into her birth position. There is very little room for her to move around in those last weeks and so she will find the most comfortable position. With the aid of gravity and the angel of your pelvis, most babies turn head down. To visualize this optimal position, imagine your baby resting on the left side of your belly, with her back curled against your belly, and facing your spine. This can cause your belly button to pop out and is a good sign that your baby is in the correct position! This position, called an OA position, which stands for occiput anterior and means that the back of her head is facing your belly. This position allows the contours of your baby's head and shoulders to most easily fit through your pelvis during labor. This position promotes a shorter, easier, and less painful labor.

Unfortunately, the lifestyle of today's mothers can include lots of sitting and resting in laid-back positions on comfy couches. When you spend a good deal of your time in these positions it often changes the way your baby rests in the womb. Due to the tilting of your pelvis in these laid-back positions, gravity pulls the heaviest parts of your baby (her back and head) towards your back instead of your belly. This is sometimes called the sunny side up position. Often mothers whose babies lie in this position experience painful back labor because they feel so much pressure on their back. This is called the OP position, which stands for occiput posterior, and means that the back of her head is facing your back.

In an optimal position, your baby's head is flexed and the average diameter of her head at your cervix is 9.4 cm, meaning you would only have to dilate to 9.4 cm to push her out. However, if your baby rests in the sunny side up position the part of her head that is facing the cervix changes. In a posterior position, the diameter of her head facing the cervix is, on average, 11.5 cm. This means you must dilate up to 2 cm more than if your baby was in an optimal position. In short, giving birth to a baby in a posterior position takes longer and is far more difficult.

You can begin to practice the positions that help your baby find her optimal position in the last six weeks of pregnancy. If you have had more than one child, the last two-to-three weeks is the recommended time for this practice. In general, you want to try and avoid positions that encourage your knees to be in a position higher than your hips, for example sitting in most office chairs. One of the worst positions for relaxing is lying back against comfy couch cushions. This enables your baby to rest against your spine, encouraging a posterior position. Alternative positions you can try while relaxing include lying on your left side, using a birth ball, leaning over cushions, sitting cross-legged on the floor, or sitting backwards on a chair with no arms and leaning forward. Place a rolled towel or wedge underneath your buttocks when you are in the car or at work, so that your knees are always lower than your pelvis. This creates the perfect angle for your baby to get in an optimal position. Also, try to not practice deep squats in yoga or exercise class until you are sure your baby is in an optimal, not posterior position. Deep squats can engage your baby into the pelvis and if your baby is posterior, she can get nestled deep into that position which makes it harder for her to turn. Try to not cross your legs, as this decreases the opening of the pelvis.

Try these exercises for at least 10 minutes a day:

Cat/Cow Modification: Get on all fours, arch your back like a cat and hold this position. Then flatten your back and feel the release. Quickly, tucking your tailbone underneath you, arch your back again. Tuck your head and tailbone and hold. Release. Repeat this ten times.

Doula Hula: Get on all fours, maintain a flat back, and imagine that you have a pencil extending from the end of your spine. Imagine drawing a figure 8 with that pencil by wiggling your tailbone. Reverse directions. Try and write your name with that pencil.

Good Dog/Bad Dog: Get on all fours and imagine you are a happy puppy. Wiggle your head and tail from side to side, trying to keep a flat back. Then abruptly, move into a "bad dog" position by tucking your bottom and head underneath, just like the cat/cow exercise. This exercise is designed to help the baby wiggle out of the pelvis and realign herself.

Open-Legged Child's Pose: Get on all fours, stretch your arms out in front of you, open your knees wide, bring your bottom towards the ground, and rest your straight arms on the floor. You can use cushions if this makes it more comfortable. You can also modify this position with a birth ball, leaning forward against the ball.

These exercises and positioning suggestions are designed to encourage your baby to get in an optimal position. Keep in mind though, every body and every baby is unique, and sometimes the best position for your baby is posterior. If your baby is posterior during labor, these exercises may encourage her to turn. For more information on positioning, please vist www.spinningbabies.com.

Common Sense Suggestions for Comfort During Labor

> *I think one of the best things we could do would be to help women/parents/families discover their own birth power, from within themselves. And to let them know it's always been there, they just needed to tap into it.*
> —John H. Kennell, MD

It is impossible to know what your labor will be like and how you will feel during your labor. Therefore, making a final decision on how you want to cope during labor is premature. What IS important is to clarify your belief system about your body, your labor, and your perception of pain. It is also critical to explore all of your options for comfort in labor. Prepare yourself with knowledge, surround yourself with the support you need, and make time to practice comfort strategies and relaxation techniques, such as deep breathing techniques and the mindful body scan. This will ensure that no matter how your labor unfolds, you will have the resources you need to cope comfortably and effectively. Preparation and the use of conscious agreement is the recipe for a positive birth experience.

This book is not designed as a childbirth manual; however, preparation for your comfort in labor starts prenatally. Here are some basic suggestions:

Prenatal Period

- Take a childbirth class that is in alignment with your belief system
- Read several good books on labor and birth
- Practice comfort strategies
- Strongly consider hiring a labor doula
- Select a place to give birth that feels good to you
- Visualize your baby
- Connect to your source
- Use conscious agreement

Labor and Birth Period

- Labor in a place that feels safe and comfortable to you
- Nourish and hydrate yourself
- Connect to your support team
- Rest/nap between contractions, use movement during contractions
- Use gravity to help your baby move down (change positions often)
- Use the tub and shower for comfort, when possible
- Use massage, hot and cold packs, aromatherapy, deep breathing techniques, or anything else that brings you comfort
- Visualize your baby
- Connect to your source
- Use conscious agreement

Please remember that this is only a very basic list of suggestions for comfort. Taking childbirth classes and hiring a doula will introduce you to a wide variety of options to increase your comfort during labor and birth.

Creating Your Labor Nest

The key to comfort in labor is creating a space, your "nest" that feels safe, private, and as homelike as possible. When you are in your nest, the instinctive part of your brain is in control, where all of your comfort hormones and labor hormones are released. The people in your nest have a significant impact on the way your labor progresses.

Decide now who will be at your labor. Birth is an exciting event and your friends and family often want to be a part of it. It's human nature to want to be close to the action. What your well-meaning friends and family do not know is that their mere presence changes the way you will labor. When you feel observed or watched, your labor hormones slow down, which means that your labor slows down too. Some people may even cause you stress, which will further inhibit your labor and reduce your ability to manage pain. Labor is designed to be a private, intimate event. When planning your support team, make certain to select only those people in your life you feel the most comfortable around.

You need to think about who will be invited to attend your labor, the birth, and the days following the birth. Make certain you communicate your wishes to everyone who potentially wants to be with you during this time. You may also want to have a plan in place to deal with uninvited visitors. Keep in mind that your support needs could change while you are in labor. Discuss this with your team now so they allow you the freedom to change your mind when necessary. Your doula or nurse can often offer suggestions if you are concerned about hurting people's feelings. Remember this is your birth. You have a right to create a sacred space to welcome your baby.

In addition to deciding who will be present for your labor, you also want to consider communicating your labor wishes to everyone on your team. This includes your partner, your doula, your midwife or OB, and other members of the healthcare team (nurse, midwife's apprentice, etc.). Traditionally, this has been done with a written birth plan. A birth plan is a written document that you create which spells out your desires during your labor and delivery, for example, "Please only discuss pain medications with me if I ask for them."

Birth plans can be useful tools for:

- Thinking about birthing options prenatally
- Clarifying your belief systems concerning your labor and delivery
- Communicating your wishes to your healthcare team *prenatally* to promote discussion
- Helping you express your values to everyone on your support team

While birth plans are useful to help clarify your birth vision prenatally, consider the following when thinking about using a birth plan at your labor:

- Sometimes birth plans can create a sense of alienation and distrust between you and your healthcare team. Some mothers write them in an effort to avoid mistreatment at the hospital. They may believe that the hospital they have chosen and/or the healthcare team they have chosen does not have their best interests at heart. Is this really the environment you want to create? Consider your objectives for writing a birth plan. Is it to communicate your wishes effectively or is it to protect yourself from choices not made in conscious agreement?
- Healthcare providers often prefer verbal communication versus written instructions. You and your partner's voices

are always more effective communication tools than a written document.

- Birth plans represent what you think you want given a certain set of circumstances you imagine for your labor and delivery. However, labor is unpredictable and is affected not only by physical circumstances, but also emotional circumstances. Many birth plans leave little room for flexibility.

- Studies show that mothers may experience a sense of failure if their birth does not go according to plan. There is no way to predict the future or know what you need until you are in that moment.

The law of attraction states that what you think about, you bring about. Birth plans are often written out of a place of fear and a desire to control the experience. You cannot control your labor and delivery any more than you can control anything in your future. What you do have control over is how you respond to your circumstances during labor.

Here are some effective tools to help you have the birth experience that you want:

- Create a vision board for your labor and delivery instead of a birth plan. Birth plans tend to focus on what you don't want while a vision board shares what you DO want.
- Have honest conversations with your healthcare providers about what you do and don't want prior to labor to help you and your healthcare team to work together more effectively.
- Carefully select your place of birth and healthcare team early in your pregnancy.
- Use conscious agreement during your labor and birth for any and all decisions. This ensures that you are making the best decisions in that moment for you and your baby based on your current circumstances.

Studies show that positive birth memories are not created by the actual events during the labor and birth, but rather how a mother felt during the birthing process. Empowerment results from conscious preparation and decision-making. Focusing on what you want and verbally communicating those desires is the best way to manifest a positive birth experience.

With each thought we have we are literally conceiving our future, and from this conception, the reality of our lives and all that we experience is born.
—Tracy Wilson Peters

Chapter 16

What's Right for Your Baby

The more people have studied different methods of bringing up children the more they have come to the conclusion that what good mothers and fathers instinctively feel like doing for their babies is the best after all.
—Benjamin Spock, Pediatrician and Child Advocate

Undoubtedly you have already been inundated with both solicited and unsolicited advice about how to raise your baby. Every day you will be faced with parenting decisions. The most important parenting decision you will ever make is the decision to trust your inner wisdom and listen to your maternal instincts. This can be challenging when the information from influential sources in your life may be in direct conflict with what you believe. This is why it is essential that conscious agreement is at the heart of every important decision you make. It always steers you down the right path.

Your maternal instincts become heightened during pregnancy. In fact, your brain actually changes to make you a better decision maker as a mother. Your sense of smell, your perception of your environment, and your ability read the expressions of others become enhanced so that you are better equipped to protect your baby. This is nature's way of protecting the human race. You are designed to be a good mother. Trust yourself.

Some common choices you might find yourself faced with in the early hours and days postpartum are breastfeeding, skin-to-skin contact, rooming in, routine medical procedures, circumcision, vaccinations, choosing a pediatrician, and unexpected occurrences. These decisions are best made prenatally so that you have the time to weigh all factors. As with every important decision that you make for yourself and your baby, it is crucial that you are in conscious agreement. Remember that the goal is to be in conscious agreement with yourself AND your baby.

Breastfeeding: Though our society tends to view breastfeeding as a choice, it is a biological need for all newborns to receive their mother's milk. Only your milk can provide the immune factors and nutrition that your baby's growing body and brain require. Breastfeeding meets all of the critical needs of your baby: warmth, nourishment, and a loving connection. The media advertises that formula (artificial milk) can provide everything that your baby needs. All of the best science today clearly shows that this is not true. Artificial milk does not contain the immune factors, enzymes, growth factors, hormones, and anti-virals (and so much more!) that help to protect, nourish and develop your baby's body and brain. Without your milk, your baby is at significant increased risk for a variety of diseases, like diabetes and allergies. Breastfeeding also protects you, the mother, from certain cancers and diseases. The decision to breastfeed will have lifelong implications for you and your baby. Preparation during pregnancy is essential to breastfeeding success. You can prepare yourself by taking a good breastfeeding class, reading about breastfeeding, going to a breastfeeding support group during pregnancy, planning to use baby-led breastfeeding techniques and talking with other mothers who have successfully breastfed.

Skin-to-Skin and Being Near Your Baby: The popularity of hospital nurseries since the 1950s has made it the norm for mothers and babies to be separated periodically in the days following birth. You and your baby need to be together. Your baby is designed to be close to you. When your baby is born, keeping her in direct skin contact (called skin-to-skin contact) actually improves her health. You might be surprised to learn that your breasts actually change temperature according to your baby's needs for warmth. Skin-to-skin contact regulates your baby's metabolism and blood sugar levels. It also helps your baby's brain stay calm, which benefits breastfeeding and overall brain growth. Research shows that when newborns are separated from their mothers, the baby's brain growth slows down and her stress levels are extremely high. Making the conscious decision to stay close to your baby not only helps you learn how to better care for and bond with your baby, but also has significant long term health benefits.

Newborn Medical Procedures: Health agencies may require that certain newborn procedures are performed on your baby, depending on the laws in your area. These can include, but are not limited to, procedures such as antibiotic eye ointment, vitamin K shots, blood tests, glucose tests, hearing tests, and genetic screening. As a parent, you should educate yourself on the benefits, risks, and legal issues surrounding these procedures by talking to your pediatrician, taking a newborn care class, and reading about newborn care. In the event that you do not feel comfortable with a certain procedure (conscious agreement), you may legally have the ability to refuse treatment by signing a waiver. You can talk to your pediatrician if you have specific questions.

Circumcision: Circumcision is a decision that some parents of male children will consider. Circumcision is the surgical removal of the foreskin from the penis. This procedure is sometimes performed for religious or cultural reasons. This decision is often very difficult for parents to make and to agree on. There is no doubt that this is a controversial topic. Due to this controversy, there has been a decade-long trend of reduced circumcision rates. Currently, only 33 percent of males are circumcised in the U.S. and only 30 percent worldwide.

Circumcision facts:

- Circumcision causes pain and physiologic stress for the newborn. Circumcision without analgesia is still practiced in the U.S. in some areas today.
- Physiologic responses to circumcision include changes in heart rate, blood pressure, oxygen saturation, and stress levels.
- Circumcised infants exhibit a stronger pain response to

subsequent routine immunization than do uncircumcised infants.

- The American Academy of Pediatrics does not recommend routine infant male circumcision.
- Circumcision can have a negative impact on the baby's ability to breastfeed in the first hours post-procedure.

Vaccines and Immunizations: For many parents, making the decision to vaccinate your child can be difficult, confusing, and even scary due to so much conflicting information. Today, more parents are refusing or delaying vaccinations for their children. The sharp increase in vaccinations given to babies, children and even teens over the last few years is a subject of great debate, to say the least. As a parent, the decision to vaccinate your child is one you should make by talking to your partner, your pediatrician, and of course by doing your own research from trusted resources.

Choosing a Pediatrician: It's wise to select a pediatrician for your baby before she arrives. Your baby's first visit with the pediatrician occurs within a few days of her birth. The last thing you will have time for in the days following the birth is interviewing and selecting the pediatrician that is right for your family. The relationship between your family and your pediatrician could potentially last for up to eighteen years, so careful selection is prudent. You will want to choose a pediatrician whose values are reflective of your own family's values. The best way to do this is to schedule an in-person interview with several pediatricians, if possible. The following are helpful questions to consider when you meet the pediatrician:

- Does your practice accept my insurance?
- (If you are a cash patient) Do you accept payment plans? Can you provide a schedule of fees for cash patients?
- Is this a solo or group practice? Who would we see if you are not available? Can I meet that person?

- What are your office hours? What happens if my child needs to be seen during the evenings or weekends?
- What hospital are you affiliated with? Will you visit my baby in the hospital after birth? If I have a homebirth, will you visit us at home?
- How does your office handle questions pertaining to my child's health that are not emergencies? Do you answer email personally?
- What are your views on breastfeeding? Circumcision? Vaccination delays and/or refusals? Babies and sleep? Antibiotics?
- What are your views on alternative or holistic models of healthcare as a complement to your care? Do you regularly refer to specific complementary practitioners, such as chiropractors or postpartum doulas?
- Does your practice employ an IBCLC (board certified lactation consultant)? If not, to whom do you refer for breastfeeding challenges?
- Does your practice give away free formula samples? (If so, this is a sign that this pediatric office may be unaware of the best ways to support breastfeeding mothers.)
- Does your practice offer educational seminars for parents?
- What parenting/baby books do you recommend?

Questions to ask yourself:

- How do I feel about the pediatrician's bedside manner?
- Does she smile?
- Is she warm?
- Do I feel comfortable with her?
- Does she seem comfortable with my baby?
- Does she interact with my baby?
- Does my baby seem comfortable with the pediatrician?
- Does she patiently respond to all of my questions?

- Does she seem well-informed and up-to-date in her thinking?
- Does she ask me how I feel about things?
- Does she seem to be respectful of my time?
- Do I feel cared for by the nurses and other staff at this practice?

Unexpected Events: Because it is impossible to know what the future holds, sometimes unexpected events arise. If you find yourself in a situation that you had not considered regarding your baby (for example, your baby needing to spend time in the intensive care nursery), it will be important to seek immediate information and resources so you are aware of all of your options. Be proactive in seeking out answers to the questions you have. In hospital settings, you can ask for the help of the patient advocate or the nurse manager for specialized situations. These individuals can help you find the support you need in any special situation. You are your baby's only voice and it is up to you to advocate for your baby, especially during unexpected events. No matter what anyone advises you to do, remember conscious agreement. Check in with your intuitive sense of what is best for you and your baby and then make a decision.

When making any decision as a parent, the most important source of information you have is always available to you and will never fail you. That source, of course, is conscious agreement.

Life After Pregnancy

The third trimester is the time to begin to prepare for what life will be like after the birth of your new baby. Making plans early for the arrival of your baby will reduce the amount of chaos you experience in those first few weeks. Many new parents are thrown off-guard by the significant transition that new parenthood brings. The reality of post-partum life is that most of your time will be spent feeding your baby, sleeping, and eating. There is not much time left over to do anything else, especially entertaining well-meaning friends and family. Gathering what you need and making decisions ahead of time will ultimately lead to less stress for your family. Less stress means a calmer baby, a more peaceful family life, better breastfeeding, more rest, improved bonding with your baby, and a faster postpartum recovery.

Nourishment: You will need to create a plan to nourish your family in the weeks that follow birth. It may seem strange now, but even preparing the smallest meal can seem overwhelming to new moms. If you are not well-nourished, then you do not have energy to care for your baby or yourself. Remember the concept of H.A.L.T and how important it is to try and minimize being hungry, angry, lonely, and tired. The nourishment cheat sheet includes:

Set up meal delivery by friends and family. There are free online programs that can help with organizing meal sign ups and deliveries. Make certain to communicate that meal delivery should not include a prolonged visit. Be sure to share any dietary restrictions or requests.

For your baby shower you can request gift cards to local restaurants that deliver food.

Ask your partner to create small snack bags or meals for you any time he plans to leave you alone with the baby.

Make meals ahead of time that can easily be frozen and warmed up when there is no time to cook. In the weeks that precede your birth, when you and your partner make dinner, simply make a double batch and freeze half of it. This is a great date night activity, creating your favorite meals together to share again when the baby is born.

Seclusion/Babymoon: The concept of the babymoon is similar to the idea of a honeymoon. You would not dream of having other people with you on your honeymoon, as it is meant to be a time to get to know one another intimately. Babymooning is meant to be a private, secluded time to get to know the new member of your family. Generally, babymooning means staying in bed, being skin-to-skin with your baby, breastfeeding on cue, eating and drinking when you want, taking lots of naps, and having private time. This means having very limited visitors. You should not have to entertain people while you are recovering from your birth and learning to breastfeed your baby. Make sure you clearly communicate this to your friends and family and tell them that you will let them know when you are ready to accept visitors. You may want to ask certain friends and family to drop off meals, do errands and light housekeeping, and help you with your new role.

Communicating Your Boundaries: Your friends and family will be excited about the new arrival of your baby and often cannot wait to meet her. This means they may drop by unexpectedly or uninvited. To help avoid these situations you can:

> Leave a note on your door indicated that you are NOT accepting visitors now, but will be accepting visitors at a later time, no exceptions.

> Change the voicemail message on your phone and/or update your social network status. The message should include all of the important information friends and family want to know about your baby, as well the fact that you are not currently accepting visitors.

> Remember that it is always okay to say no. You can ask that visitors come back at a later time, when invited. You can also share with them that most healthcare

providers suggest that babies are not exposed to anyone but the family for the first weeks postpartum.

Housework: Have a discussion with your partner now about housework. It is impossible to care for the baby, yourself, AND do housework in early weeks of your baby's life. Decide now what critical tasks must be done every day, such as dishes and laundry, and let the rest go. Consider easy ways to get these jobs accomplished.

Consider paper plates and disposable utensils in the fist few days.

Often friends and family really want to help, but don't know what to do. Make a list of the things you need done and ask them to pick something to do off of your list.

Ask for money to go towards a month of maid service at your baby shower. You can also save a few dollars a week throughout your pregnancy to go towards this expense.

The Ideal Nest: You probably have spent months decorating your nursery. The reality is that most families spend very little time in the nursery. Babies are meant to be near their mothers. Make no mistake; a baby monitor does not substitute for your presence. While monitors allow you to hear your baby's cry, crying is a late sign of distress and hunger. The American Academy of Pediatrics recommends that breastfeeding babies sleep in close proximity to their mothers. All babies, whether they are breastfed or bottle fed, benefit from sleeping near their mother. Keeping your baby near you during sleeping times means that you will want to create a safe space for your baby to sleep. If you want more information on creating a safe co-sleeping space, look for resources and books from Dr. James McKenna. Choose one or two easily accessible rooms that you plan on spending most of your time in and make sure they are well-stocked with items you and your baby will need (diapers, water, snacks, breast pads, etc.).

Postpartum help: The following is a list of professionals/groups that can help you in the weeks following the birth. It is helpful to know how to find them before your baby arrives.

> Lactation consultants: These professionals can help you if you experience challenges with breastfeeding. They should have the credential IBCLC, which stands for International Board Certified Lactation Consultant. They can often be found at the hospital, pediatric offices, or in private practice.

> La Leche League: This free mother-to-mother support group has been supporting breastfeeding moms since the 1950s. Mothers are encouraged to attend the group meetings even during pregnancy to meet other mothers and become familiar with the league leaders. You can find a list of meetings near you on the La Leche League website.

> Postpartum doulas: These doulas specialize in supporting families in the home after the birth. It is important to interview and hire a postpartum doula well before the baby arrives. Often, postpartum doulas are booked well in advance because they tend to work with only a few families at a time. You can find postpartum doulas on the CAPPA, DONA, and ICEA websites.

> Car seat technicians: These professionals train parents how to safely install a car seat in their vehicle. This short training is crucial to the safety of your child, as the majority of car seats are installed incorrectly, which can lead to a

major injury and/or death in the event of a car accident. Often car seat training is provided free of charge by community organizations. Some fire stations, hospitals, and motor vehicle departments employ or offer resources for car seat technicians. Make certain to take part in this training before your baby arrives.

New mother/breastfeeding support groups: Be aware of the multitude of new mother support groups that are available to you in your area. These can often be found at hospitals, baby stores, WIC (Women Infants Children) offices, churches, libraries, and community centers. There are groups that offer support for different needs, including mothers of multiples, breastfeeding, postpartum depression, back to work, and special needs babies. There are even groups just for dads.

Siblings: Some mothers have fears that they will not be able to love a new baby as much as they love their first child. While your relationship with your new baby will be different, there is no reason to worry that there is not enough love to go around. Love is limitless and there are no boundaries to this emotion. However, don't expect your relationship with the new baby to be the same as the relationship with your first. Every baby is a unique individual and your relationship will develop over time, just as it did with your first child. If you are concerned about this, it may be comforting to talk to mothers who have more than one child about their experiences. Just as you will develop a new relationship with your baby, her siblings will also need time to make the transition. While exciting, becoming a big brother or sister can be overwhelming for some children. Here are some suggestions to help make this transition easier:

Celebrate becoming a big brother or sister. Having a new baby is also rite of passage for your child. Small gestures can go a long way towards making your child feel more included and important in their new role as big brother or sister. You and your partner can research and decide on some specific ways you can honor this new role for your child. For example, some families have a special big brother or sister party before the birth to celebrate this special transition and new role for their child.

Have your children attend the birth of their new brother or sister. It can be a meaningful experience for everyone. If your child wants to be present and you are comfortable having him/her at the birth, you should prepare them for what they might see and hear in advance. It can be scary for your child to see you in pain or hear you make unfamiliar noises. Keep in mind that you and your partner will not have the capacity at some points in labor to comfort and care for their needs. This means that all young children present at birth should have their own support person to care for them. Careful preparation ahead of time can make the birth of the new baby a joyful experience for the entire family.

Find a sibling class to teach your child how to safely interact with the new baby. These classes are designed to make your child feel special while also helping to set up safe boundaries for interacting with their new brother or sister. Additionally, you can find many movies and books on becoming a big brother or sister at your local library or on the internet.

Plan special time with your older child. Make a conscious effort to create one-on-one time with your older child every day. While you and your partner may find that you may initially have limited opportunities to do this, you can ask other family members and friends to step in and give your child extra love and attention. Try and set up short play dates for your child as often as possible after the baby arrives.

Make breastfeeding a special time for everyone. You can make breastfeeding "family time" by planning activities for your older child in advance. An example of this might include offering special snacks, books, or toys that are only brought out while you are breastfeeding. Keep in mind that some previously weaned toddlers may display a renewed interest in breastfeeding. This is normal and natural behavior and something to consider before the baby arrives.

Pets: You will need to consider your pet's potential reaction to your new baby. Pets can be unpredictable. Even the most trusted and loving animals can display aggression, assertive behavior or playful behavior than can accidentally harm your baby. Be aware of unexpected and/or potentially dangerous reactions to your baby. There are often community classes for families who will be bringing a new baby into a home with pets. You can typically find these at large veterinary practices, animal shelters, and pet stores. These classes will offer you many options to help keep your baby and your pet safe. If classes are not available, you can find plenty of internet resources on the topic. Injuries to your baby can occur unintentionally, even when your animal isn't being aggressive, such as scratches. Careful and constant supervision of all pets allowed near your baby is strongly urged. It may take weeks or longer for your pets to adapt to your baby. Some pets may never adapt and may need to be kept separate from your baby. Be aware that animals, especially cats, can jump into your baby's bed and are often attracted to the scent of a baby. This should not be allowed as it could injure your baby. If your baby is left in a crib, make sure you keep the door closed so that animals cannot access her room or crib. There is also a possibility that your baby could have an allergy to your pets, though some research suggests that early exposure to pets reduces the risk of dander allergies. Be sure to mention your pets to your pediatrician if your baby shows any symptoms of an allergic response.

Let's talk about sex: Things will change. Your body will change. Your time and energy resources will change. Your relationship with your partner will change. These changes bring both challenges and opportunities for your relationship. You will need to find new definitions for intimacy. Generally, during the first six weeks postpartum, sexual intercourse is not recommended because your body is healing from the birth process. However, intimacy is well advised. Cuddling, hugging, kissing, and snuggling all can help you and your partner stay connected. Things to consider when you are ready to resume intercourse:

> Birth control: While the act of breastfeeding can suppress your ability to conceive, it is not a guarantee that you will not get pregnant. If you wish to forgo traditional birth control, make sure that you are aware of the Lactation Amenorrhea Method (LAM). You can find many resources on how to utilize this method in books and online. Your healthcare provider can suggest a safe means of birth control that is compatible with breastfeeding. Make certain that you have a birth control plan in place *before* you resume sexual intercourse.

> Hormones and your postpartum body: Your hormones make a huge shift post pregnancy. These hormonal changes can cause vaginal dryness, decreased sex drive, and breast tenderness. Additionally, many women experience soreness and swelling in the perineum and

vaginal area. Some women may also be recovering from a cesarean section, a perineal tear, or an episiotomy. This can make the thought of having sex again a little frightening. Careful planning before resuming sexual intercourse can make the experience less stressful and more enjoyable. Be sure you plan for enough time and privacy, and make sure you have any products you might need, such as lubricant.

Communication: Have open and honest conversations with your partner about one another's feelings regarding sex and intimacy. Don't assume that your partner understands what your body is going through, or that you understand his needs either. Communication is key to the health of your relationship. Both partners have needs that are important. If you ignore one another's needs, it becomes more and more difficult as time passes to maintain a healthy relationship. Discuss ways that you both can have your intimacy needs met, even when you may be tired and time is tight. Be creative, intimacy isn't just sex.

Birth is not only about making babies. Birth is about making mothers...strong, competent, capable mothers who trust themselves and know their inner strength.
—Barbara Katz Rothman

With all of the decisions that you will need to make, it is easy to feel overwhelmed. Fortunately, you do not need to make all final decisions right now. Now is the time to consider all of your options, talk with your partner and use conscious agreement as you prepare to become a new family.

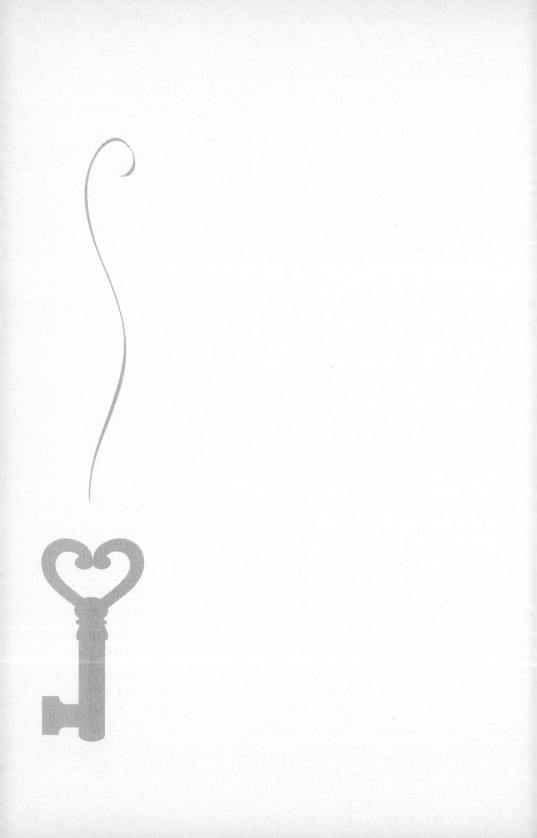

Chapter Seventeen

Keys to Selecting the Birth Place

Where will you have your baby?

There are many options for the place of birth and not one place is right for every mother. The vast majority of women in the U.S., well over ninety percent, will give birth in the hospital, although home-births and birth center births have recently been on the rise. Each option for birth has advantages and disadvantages, so use careful consideration and conscious agreement to make this important decision.

Before you consider where you will give birth, you should take into consideration where you might be most comfortable. It may sound strange to hear the words "comfortable" and "birth" linked together, but your comfort has a significant impact on how you will labor and birth. Your comfort isn't only related to the physical sensations in labor; it is also about your feelings of safety, support, and overall well-being. Your body is always eavesdropping on your thoughts. This will be true during your labor and birth, thus the importance of feeling safe and supported during the process.

If you are scared, without the support you need, or otherwise stressed your thoughts will reflect these feelings and your body may respond by slowing the labor progress. Stress during labor can also increase the perception of pain. Stress hormones are shared with the baby. At times, unresolved stress can cause fetal distress, which in turn, can lead to unnecessary interventions or surgery. Choosing the place where you will give birth is a very personal decision. Not everyone feels comfortable or safe in a hospital, just as not everyone would feel comfortable giving birth at home. This decision is about *you* and where *you* feel safe.

Many families desire the warmth, comfort, and relaxed, family-focused environment that a homebirth provides. While hospitals have taken great strides in trying to emulate the look of home, the décor of the hospital has nothing to do with the type of "care" you will receive there. Do not expect a homebirth experience if you plan to give birth in a hospital. Alternatively, do not expect a homebirth to offer what a hospital has.

BABY-FRIENDLY FACILITIES

According to Baby-Friendly® USA, "baby-friendly facilities have taken special steps to create the best possible environment for successful breastfeeding." These facilities have implemented the Ten Steps to Successful Breastfeeding that have been recommended by the World Health Organization and UNICEF. These steps include:

1. Have a written breastfeeding policy that is routinely communicated to all healthcare staff.

2. Train all healthcare staff in skills necessary to implement this policy.

3. Inform all pregnant women about the benefits and management of breastfeeding.

4. Help mothers initiate breastfeeding within an hour of birth.

5. Show mothers how to breastfeed and how to maintain lactation, even if they should be separated from their infants.

6. Give newborn infants no food or drink other than breast milk, unless medically indicated.

7. Practice "rooming in" by allowing mothers and infants to remain together 24 hours a day.

8. Encourage breastfeeding on demand.

9. Give no artificial nipples, pacifiers, dummies, or soothers to breastfeeding infants.

10. Foster the establishment of breastfeeding support groups and refer mothers to them on discharge from the hospital or birthing center.

These steps can be found at http://www.unicef.org/programme/breastfeeding/baby.htm.

You can get more information at www.babyfriendlyusa.org.

MOTHER-FRIENDLY CARE

The Coalition for Improved Maternity Services sponsors an initiative that is designed to support the philosophical cornerstones of mother-friendly care. These cornerstones include normalcy of the birthing process, empowerment, autonomy, do no harm, and responsibility. A mother-friendly facility agrees to do the following:

Offers all birthing mothers:

- Unrestricted access to the birth companions of her choice;
- Unrestricted access to continuous emotional and physical support from a skilled professional;
- Access to professional midwifery care.

- Provides accurate descriptive and statistical information to the public about its practices and procedures for birth care, including measures of interventions and outcomes.
- Provides culturally competent care.
- Provides the birthing woman with the freedom to walk, move about, and assume the positions of her choice during labor and birth (unless restriction is specifically required to correct a complication), and discourages the use of the lithotomy position.
- Has clearly defined policies and procedures for: collaborating and consulting throughout the perinatal period with other maternity services, including communicating with the original caregiver when transfer from one birth site to another is necessary; linking the mother and baby to appropriate community resources, including prenatal and post-discharge follow-up and breastfeeding support.
- Does not routinely employ practices and procedures that are unsupported by scientific evidence.
- Has a VBAC (vaginal birth after cesarean) rate of 60% or more with a goal of 75% or more.
- Educates staff in non-drug methods of pain relief, and does not promote the use of analgesic or anesthetic drugs not specifically required to correct a complication.
- Encourages all mothers and families, including those with sick or premature newborns or infants with congenital problems, to touch, hold, breastfeed, and care for their babies to the extent compatible with their conditions.
- Discourages non-religious circumcision of the newborn.
- Strives to achieve the WHO-UNICEF "Ten Steps of the Baby-Friendly Hospital Initiative" to promote successful breastfeeding.

© 1996 Coalition for Improving Maternity Services (CIMS)
You can get more information at motherfriendly.org.

The healthcare provider that you chose to support you at birth will play a part in where you have your baby. So how do you go about making this decision?

If you have a midwife as your provider, your possible options can include a hospital birth, birth center, or homebirth dependant on how she practices. If you have a physician or obstetrician, it is most likely that she only offers care in a hospital setting. Some obstetricians work in free-standing birth centers alongside midwives, but it is still a rare occurrence in the United States. Often obstetricians will have practicing privileges at several hospital locations, so it is up to you to do your homework to determine which hospital is the best fit for your family if you choose an obstetrician or physician as your provider.

Questions to ask the hospital:

- Do you offer private rooms for labor and delivery and post-partum?
- Do you have restrictions on who can support me during labor? Partner? Doula? Family members? Is there a limit on the number of people who can be in the room?
- What percentage of births are first time cesarean deliveries? What percentage are repeat cesarean deliveries?
- What are my options for pain relief? What non-medicated comfort strategies do you offer? (Birth balls, music, aromatherapy, shower/tub, etc.) Is unmedicated birth supported? If I choose anesthesia, is there an anesthesiologist available around the clock? Are there any limitations on when I can have an epidural?
- How many patients does each nurse take care of at the same time?
- Is this hospital mother-friendly? Is this hospital baby-friendly?
- Are there routine procedures that I must accept as part of labor? (Examples include having an IV, continuous monitoring, and confinement to bed.)

- Is this hospital equipped to deal with emergencies in the event that they arise? When might a mother or baby be transferred from this facility?
- Can I eat during my labor?
- Can I take pictures or videos of my labor and birth? What if I have a cesarean?
- Once I check into the facility as a patient, do I have to have my baby within a certain period of time before medical intervention occurs, provided mother and baby are fine?
- What are my options for delivery? Do you offer waterbirth?
- Does the hospital encourage skin-to-skin care at birth and throughout the hospital stay?
- How does the hospital support breastfeeding? Does the hospital offer breastfeeding support in the form of lactation consulting?
- Does the hospital keep mothers and babies together continuously, or offer rooming in? What are the reasons my baby might be separated from me?
- Are babies given pacifiers if they are breastfed? (Pacifier use in the first four weeks postpartum can negatively impact breastfeeding success in health full term babies.)
- What is the hospital policy on formula supplementation for breastfed babies?
- Does the hospital have a neonatal intensive care unit? What level of care do they offer?
- How long will I stay in the hospital after the birth of my baby with a vaginal birth? With a cesarean birth?
- What precautions do you have in place to prevent infant abduction and infant switching?
- What routine medical procedures are required for my baby at this hospital?
- Who can stay with me after the birth? What are you visitation policies?

This may seem like an overwhelming list of questions to ask the hospital. However, you should keep in mind that hospitals are designed to provide medical care for the masses. They are not designed for individualized care. They have many policies and procedures in place to protect their patients and the hospital staff, which can impact individual freedoms. Hospitals are designed to treat people during illness and emergencies, not necessarily to protect the individual emotional needs and well-being of mothers, babies, and families. It is up to you to be your own advocate at a hospital and surround yourself with a support team who will tend to your emotional needs.

Your insurance, or lack thereof, may also be a consideration. Some policies dictate not only where you give birth but the type of care provider you must use. Not all insurance policies will allow you the option to select a midwife as a care provider or to give birth at a birth center or at home instead of a hospital. If you do not have insurance coverage then cost may be a factor for you. If cost is an issue for you, many practitioners have payment plans.

Where you give birth should ultimately be based on where you feel the safest and most comfortable. Whether you choose the hospital, birth center, or your home, it is important that you can create a space, your "nest," where you and your partner feel secure. Mammals have the most successful births when they are in an undisturbed atmosphere of privacy and intimacy. For example, have you ever observed a pet in labor? Did you notice that she chose the darkest, quietest, most secluded space she could find to labor in? Animals seek privacy and seclusion when in labor. In fact, it's common that mammals will completely stop their labor if disturbed. Human beings are no exception.

Hospitals frequently encounter women who arrive at the hospital with slowed or stalled contractions, although they had experienced strong and frequent contractions at home. This is due to fact that they have left their "nest" or place of comfort and the rush to the hospital can create worry, anxiety, and stress. These stress hormones reduce the body's ability to labor. Nature is intelligent in its design to protect the baby. If a mother perceives stress and becomes fearful, her body slows labor to protect the baby from being born in a dangerous environment. Unfortunately, many things in our world create a stress response for the human mother. This is why you want to choose a place to labor and birth that feels safe and secure.

When a mother labors, her mammalian brain is releasing all of the hormones necessary to give birth: oxytocin (the contraction hormone), progesterone (the cervical softening hormone), and beta-endorphins (comfort hormones). The mammalian brain is known as the instinctive brain and works best when the thinking brain (neocortex) is not being stimulated. Things that activate the thinking brain are bright lights, loud or disruptive noises, the feeling of being observed or watched, unwanted touch or intrusion, the sense of danger, or any situation that requires active decision-making. Once the thinking brain is engaged you are more likely to release stress hormones, such as adrenaline and catecholamines. Stress hormones in early and active labor interfere with the brain's release of oxytocin, which is necessary for a productive labor.

Ashley's Story

Ashley and Jonathan have prepared for their birth for many months: taking childbirth classes, hiring a doula, practicing relaxation techniques at home, and selecting the place of birth that felt best to them. It was 2 PM when Ashley had her first real contraction. She immediately called Jonathan and they decided to meet at home. Together, they labored for hours. Jonathan massaged Ashley's back, offered her tea, and timed the contractions. He made her one of her favorite light meals and played music from her specially selected playlist for her labor.

Ana, their doula, arrived around 10 PM. Both Ashley and Jonathan were glad to see her. Secretly, Jonathan was surprised how long labor was lasting. Ana knew just what to do and headed straight to the bathroom to draw a warm bath and light candles to create a safe and comfortable space. Once Ashley got in the bath, surrounded by her husband and doula, her contractions got stronger, longer, and closer together. Even though her labor became more intense, she was not afraid because she felt safe and secure with her birth team. The three of them sat in the warm glow of the candles, as Ashley rocked back and forth in the water. Jonathan noticed that Ashley's contractions were coming closer together and she was beginning to moan with each one. Within thirty minutes, Ashley looked at Jonathan with tears of excitement and said, "I think it's time to go."

Immediately, Jonathan's mind focused on getting the car ready and he tried to remember where he had to park at the hospital. He felt shaky with anticipation and was immediately grateful he had Ana there to help while he got everything ready. As Jonathan warmed up the car, in his excitement he sent an innocent text message to his sister saying, "It's time!" Little did Jonathan know, this message was immediately forwarded to his mother, Joan. His mother decided she couldn't wait at home as planned and headed directly to the hospital.

Back inside, Ana grabbed a warm towel from the dryer to wrap around Ashley and then helped her get dressed. Ana prepared Ashley for the ride by giving her an eye mask, headphones with her favorite music playing, a stress ball to squeeze, and a warm heat pack for her back. Ana knew these techniques would help keep Ashley in her "nest" for the drive to the hospital, twenty minutes away. Once she had Ashley settled in the car with Jonathan, Ana said she would see them soon and drove separately to the hospital.

At the hospital, Jonathan dropped off Ashley with the hospital attendant and sped away to park the car. Ashley was placed in a wheelchair, whisked up an elevator to the labor and delivery floor, and situated in her birthing room. She started to feel anxious and wondered where her doula and husband were. After the nurse had finished asking Ashley what seemed like hundreds of medical questions, she handed Ashley a plastic cup and a hospital gown and asked her to give a urine sample and get changed. Ashley noticed that, strangely, her contractions had slowed down but felt much more painful.

In the bathroom, Ashley began to cry. She had only been alone for ten minutes, but it seemed like the longest ten minutes of her life. Finally, she heard a soft knock at the door and it was Jonathan. Ashley embraced him and began to cry harder, asking, "Where have you been all of this time and where's Ana?" Before Jonathan could answer, the nurse walked into the bathroom and said, "Let's get you on the monitor and see how that baby is doing." Ashley got into the hospital bed and her nurse placed the monitors on her belly. Ashley was uncomfortable and found that both her position in the bed and the placement of the monitors increased the pain in her back.

Ana arrived, introduced herself to the nurse and immediately began massaging Ashley's feet, as she knew this would help comfort her. The nurse told them she would leave now and return in a while to check the monitor. Noticing Ashley's pain, Ana asked the nurse if it would be okay to have Ashley labor on the birthing ball while she was being monitored. The nurse agreed and helped Ashley onto the ball before she left the room. Ana showed Jonathan where to massage Ashley's back and she turned down the lights and played some soft music. As Ashley relaxed on the ball, she leaned forward to rest on the hospital bed. Ana placed Ashley's pillow from home under her head and the smell of home immediately relaxed her. Ashley began to feel more comfortable in her surroundings and started to rock on the birthing ball. Ana massaged Ashley's hands and the three of them settled into this new nest they had created at the hospital. After some time, Jonathan noticed that the contractions on the monitor screen were coming more frequently. He told Ashley, "It won't be long now, honey, things have picked back up."

Just then, the nurse came into the room with Jonathan's mother, Joan, in tow. Everyone was surprised to see Joan, as she had been asked to stay at home until the baby arrived. Even though Ashley was irritated by Joan's arrival, she did not want to say anything to hurt her mother-in-law's feelings. "Why is it so dark in here?" Joan asked as she turned on the lights. She then walked over to Ashley and asked her numerous questions, and shared details of her own long and painful labors. Joan handed Jonathan a dollar bill and asked him to get her a cup of coffee, since it was going to be a long night. Jonathan reluctantly complied.

During Jonathan's absence, Joan continued to chatter which made it difficult for Ashley to concentrate on her contractions. Ana noticed that Ashley's contractions were again slowing down and yet her pain level was increasing. Joan's presence was obviously disrupting the safe and secure nest they had created. When Jonathan returned, Ana took him to the side and quietly mentioned that Ashley seemed to need more privacy than she currently had. Jonathan agreed and asked Ana for a suggestion on how to handle this delicate situation. They decided it would be a good idea to send Joan on some important errands that would keep her busy for a couple of hours or more.

Once Joan hesitantly left, Ana suggested that Ashley try laboring in the tub again, since that worked so well at home. Ashley liked this idea. Jonathan and Ana worked together to support Ashley while she labored in the tub. Ashley's labor quickly progressed in the more intimate environment. Her baby was born in the early morning and Joan and the rest of the family arrived to welcome the new family member. Later in the day, as Ashley held her baby, she reflected back on her birth experience. She told Jonathan that what seemed to work best for her labor was the intimate, loving support that he and Ana offered her. She expressed her gratitude to Jonathan. She also shared that she realized she was happy to have the entire family there after the baby arrived. This was an important lesson for Ashley and Jonathan as parents, to learn that trusting their instincts and following through with them was always the right decision.

This segment contains information that can help you make a decision on where you want to give birth. Remember to not only consider the pros and cons but also how the idea of laboring at each location makes you *feel*. Ideally, the place of birth needs to be considered very early on in pregnancy (much earlier than the third trimester). However, if you find at any point that you are no longer in conscious agreement with your previously chosen place of birth, it is within your power to change your mind.

CONSCIOUS AGREEMENT CONSIDERATIONS

SAFETY

Hospital Birth
Access to immediate emergency services, medications, operating room, and potential access to neonatal intensive care unit.

Birth Center
Close proximity to emergency services, medications, and operating room

Homebirth
Proximity to emergency services, medications and an operating room is dependent on the location of the home. Data shows that most homebirths have low rates of transfers to hospital and lower risk of cesarean section and medical intervention.

COMFORT

Hospital Birth
While you may have access to both medical and non-medical pain relief, consider that hospitals can limit your ability to move, restrict intake of food, and may

not allow use of the tub or shower. Hospitals utilize medical equipment and have policies in place that can interfere with your comfort and endorphin release.

Birth Center

You will have access to many natural comfort strategies in a birth center. However, there may or may not be access to pain medications. Most birth centers offer continuous labor support, which can contribute to your comfort and endorphin release. Many birth centers offer both hydrotherapy and waterbirth options.

Homebirth

When you are home, you are in an environment that you have created. You are surrounded by the people, smells, sights, and things that you are most familiar with. You have the freedom to choose the support you want, when and where you want it. You have complete control over your environment, from what you wear to what you eat to who surrounds you. Ask your midwife about access to pain medications, if that is important to you.

ATTENDANTS

Hospital Birth

While you will be able to choose your personal support team, the hospital may restrict the overall number of people supporting you. Children may be discouraged from attending or not be permitted at all. Additionally, you may have very little control over who your healthcare team is, including your doctor.

Birth Center

Most birth centers tend to be more flexible in allowing you to choose your birth team. Check with your local birth center about visitation policies.

Homebirth

You get to choose all of your attendants at your birth. There are no restrictions. Check with your midwife to see who her backup or assistant will be.

NOURISHMENT/ HYDRATION

Hospital Birth

Hospitals often have policies that restrict nourishment during labor. This has been shown to have a negative impact on labor and the perception of pain. Use of intravenous fluids (I.V.) is commonplace in hospitals.

Birth Center

You are encouraged to eat and drink as you wish throughout labor.

Homebirth

Not only can you eat and drink when you wish at home, but you are surrounded by the foods and drinks that you enjoy. You also have people around you who can cook meals as needed.

PRIVACY

Hospital Birth

You will have very little privacy at the hospital. You do not get to choose who comes in your room, or even when they come in (with the exception of you own birth team).

Birth Center

While you may have more privacy at a birth center than at a hospital, there still may be times that your privacy is compromised.

Homebirth

It's your home, you decide the level of privacy that you need and have ultimate control over your environment. For example, you may have several friends present in your house during your labor, but you may choose to go to another room.

MEDICAL PROCEDURES

Hospital Birth

Medical technologies and procedures carry both benefits and risks. At the hospital, many routine medical policies and procedures are standard, some of which may not be medically necessary for your individualized care. Familiarize yourself with the routine procedures and be certain to take a hospital tour and ask the questions mentioned in this chapter. By talking to your care provider, you may be able to avoid unnecessary procedures. More than a third of all U.S. women who give birth in a hospital give birth via cesarean section.

Birth Center

Most medical procedures encountered at birth centers are not routine, but instead are available in the event that they become necessary. Take a tour of your birth center and ask questions about their medical procedures and policies.

Homebirth

The medical procedures that are available at a homebirth are often determined by state laws, and by the type of care provider attending the birth. In the event of an emergency or required cesarean, you will need to be transferred to the hospital. The distance between your home and the nearest hospital should be taken into consideration.

RECORDING YOUR BIRTH

Hospital Birth

Many hospitals have restrictions on still photography, as well as video recording. Check with the hospital and your care provider about their policies.

Birth Center

It is uncommon for birth centers to place restriction on photography or video recording. However, to be sure, check with your birth center.

Homebirth

You can record anything you wish at a homebirth. It is your home and your birth. Check with your midwife to make sure she has no objections.

COST

Hospital Birth

Hospitals accept most insurance policies. If you are not covered by an insurance policy, check with the hospital about cash payment options. Consider all the fees associated with hospital birth, including the doctor/pediatrician fees, lab fees, anesthesia cost, medication, etc.

Birth Center

Some birth centers accept certain insurance plans. However, it is likely that you may need to pay out of pocket for some or all of your care. Check with the birth center.

Homebirth

The majority of homebirth care is done on a cash basis, and often includes your prenatal care with your midwife as part of the package. There may be limited insurance coverage, check with your insurance provider. It is common in the U.S. for homebirths to be less than one quarter the cost of a vaginal hospital birth.

Where you choose to give birth will affect how you labor. If you do plan on a hospital birth, doula care is especially helpful, as it is unlikely that you will have continuous support from the medical staff.

⚷ Master Keys – Tips From the Experts

Selecting a doula to be part of your team can benefit your labor and birth in so many ways. This interview with Polly Perez, a leader and mentor in the doula profession for the past forty years, explains the role of doulas and how they can positively impact birth. Mrs. Perez is a perinatal nurse, doula, childbirth educator, and the author of *Special Women: The Role of the Professional Labor Assistant* and *The Nurturing Touch: A Labor Support Handbook*.

Mrs. Perez answered the following questions:

Why should a mother consider hiring a doula?

"All laboring women deserve to be nurtured, loved, attended to, and supported as they undertake the journey to the birth of their child. That journey can be one of the most life-changing experiences of their lives. I have always felt that the best answer to this question came from a mother herself when she said to me, 'My doula was my friend, my strength, my shield, my teacher, and, most of all, my anchor in a sea of confusion, pain, and fatigue. She was to me what a lighthouse was to a ship, a gentle guide showing you your destination and helping you avoid unnecessary hazards.'"

How do doulas benefit babies?

"Doulas help babies by helping their mothers listen and trust their instincts. This helps mothers bond with their babies, respond to their babies, and love them unconditionally."

What makes a great doula?

"The attributes I would encourage you to look for in a doula center around the emotional spectrum: a caring heart, loyalty, respect for you and your partner as individuals, listening to your needs and wants, and believing in you even when you don't believe in yourself."

What is the most important thing to know when hiring a doula?

"The most important thing is to interview several doulas before picking one. You want to find the best doula for you, individually."

Do women who plan on having an epidural need a doula?

"Even though you might be planning to have a epidural, you will definitely still benefit by having the services of a doula. Your doula will be there to nurture you, comfort you, and support you and your birth choices regardless of your pain relief choices. She will be there continually, help explain what is happening to you, help you change positions so that your labor will progress, help you advocate for yourself; and, if the need arises, she will pull out many doula "tricks of the trade" that will help you physically and emotionally. Even though you have chosen analgesia for your labor, you will still need and want emotional support. The doula will continue to put your needs and wants in the forefront. She will focus of what you are thinking and feeling emotionally. Your partner will also benefit from the services of a doula, as she will support your partner in supporting you. The doula will give both of you the reassurance and support you need for you to have a positive birth memory."

You mentioned that partners benefit from a doula. How so?

"I had been working as a childbirth educator and perinatal nurse for many years and then in the early 1980s, I had two different men ask me to personally be at their children's births for THEM. As they said, 'I want you to help me help her through the whole labor and delivery.' These men introduced me to what I now call doula-dom. People always assume that I got into this doula profession because of the mothers, but in my case it was really because of the fathers. I started to focus on the dads so that they could focus on concentrating on the needs and wants of their partner. A good doula doesn't replace the dad; we are there to back him up. We can give him hints, advice, and reminders that he can use to help his partner. The doula can easily speak 'hospital-eze' and translate it into more readily understood terms. She can encourage a father to participate as he and his partner want or need. If a father doesn't want to take an active role, he can be assured that his partner is still getting one-on-one support by the doula. Some men want to simply experience the birth on their own terms.

The doula also knows what questions to ask. A doula can never replace the father's role, which is to love and support his partner, because doulas are not the father of this baby. Yes, we know many 'tricks of the trade,' but the father knows his partner far better than we do. Part of our job is be a back-up to him and be sure that he has drinks and snacks so he can keep his energy up during the labor and birth. The father and the doula often can tag-team, if needed or wanted. The doula's presence allows the father to take the guilt-free breaks he often needs. Sometime the father wants only to hold his partner's hand and give her verbal encouragement while the doula takes a more active role. This team approach allows the mother to feel continually supported and cared for by both of them. Dads and doulas make a wonderful team!"

For more information on doulas, read Mrs. Perez's book, *Special Women*. To find a doula, contact **CAPPA, DONA or ICEA.**

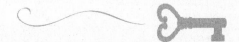

Chapter Eighteen

Keys to Physical Support in the Third Trimester

"If you let go of fear, fear will let go of you."
—Unknown

Your last trimester is a time of incredible growth, physically, emotionally, and spiritually. A transformation is occurring. You are transforming into a new you. For most women this change does not come without some fear and anxiety. Fear and worry are part of the mothering process. The concerns that arise are, in fact, blessings for you and your baby. These brilliantly disguised gifts of worry provide a way for you to begin to address the things in your life that need attention. This is nature's way of helping you become the best mother you can be. In fact, in the last weeks of pregnancy, your brain naturally begins to release small levels of the stress hormone cortisol. This helps you to become a more protective and attentive mother by being more aware of your surroundings. It also intensifies any feelings of worry you might have.

Allow yourself to fully experience these feelings of fear and worry. Exploring them and coming to peace with them will ultimately result in more confident mothering. This does not mean that you will eliminate your fears, simply that you become mindful of them. This reduces the power that fear has over you and your life. Pushing fear away prevents you from facing issues that you intuitively *know* might interfere with the motherbaby bond. Not only can repressed fear manifest as emotional discomfort, it can also increase physical discomforts. Remember that your body is always listening in on your thoughts. Any disturbance in your emotional health can result in physical symptoms. When you experience a physical discomfort, begin first by checking in with your emotions and thoughts.

Third Trimester Physical Changes

Important Note: Always check with your healthcare provider about the safety and efficacy of any treatment for your personal situation.

Fluid Retention: Your body is processing more fluid and makes more blood during pregnancy, which often results in swelling or edema. In fact, up to a quarter of your pregnancy weight can be due to this excess fluid. In the last trimester of pregnancy, it is common to begin to notice even more swelling as your growing baby can put excess pressure on your veins. You might find that your fingers, feet, and ankles, and even your face, can feel swollen. The annoyance of edema is easier to accept once you realize that it helps with the softening of your joints and tissues to prepare for birth. While edema is common, you want to be careful that the swelling is not excessive or comes on quickly with other symptoms such as dizziness, headache, or blurry vision, which can indicate something more serious like pre-eclampsia. Call your healthcare provider if you notice the symptoms just mentioned. Keep in mind the following if you experience edema:

- Hydrate. While it might seem counterintuitive, your body needs water to process fluids. Avoid drinks with caffeine and high sodium, as they can contribute to swelling. Salting your food to taste is fine. Avoid eating salty foods, especially processed foods that contain high levels of sodium.
- Focus on foods that are high in potassium. Great examples include bananas, dates, beans, seeds (pumpkin and sunflower, though choose unsalted versions), unsalted pistachios, avocados, and surprise: chocolate!

- Try not to stand for long periods of time. Take breaks as often as possible and elevate your feet when you can.
- Get moving! Exercise helps your circulation. Swimming is especially helpful.
- Get a prenatal massage. Massage can help your body process fluids.

Heartburn: Remember the hormone relaxin that does so much to help soften your ligaments so you can deliver your baby? Relaxin also works on the valve at the esophagus, which means stomach acid can escape and cause uncomfortable heartburn. While heartburn may be an issue that you experience throughout pregnancy, it typically becomes aggravated during the third trimester as your growing baby also puts pressure on the stomach. This discomfort can be experienced after meals, during stress or emotional upset, and also can be related to food allergies or candidiasis (yeast infection). You can try using the techniques that follow to minimize the irritation of heartburn. If you continue to experience heartburn that does not resolve quickly or is very painful, contact your healthcare provider.

- Eat smaller meals more frequently. Chew your food completely before swallowing. Stretch after meals and try not to recline for at least an hour after a meal.
- Avoid caffeinated drinks, as they can increase heartburn symptoms. Try comforting, digestion supportive teas such as chamomile, fennel, lemon verbena, peppermint, and licorice *after* meals. Drinking large amounts of fluids with meals dilutes the digestive enzymes that help to process your meal.
- Spice up your meals with herbs that support healthy digestion. This includes ginger, anise seed, fennel bulb, caraway seed, peppermint, and dill weed.
- Try tissue salts. The remedy natrum mur (chloride of sodium) is commonly used to treat heartburn. This remedy can be helpful due to the imbalance of tissue salts in the

body during pregnancy. The demands of the placenta and increased fluid and blood can cause slight imbalances. Tissue salts can be found in most health food stores. Check with your healthcare provider for the best dosage.

- Homeopathy is often a safe and effective way to treat many pregnancy symptoms, including heartburn. You can find homeopathic remedies in vitamin or natural food stores. Common homeopathic treatments for heartburn include carbo veg, nux vomica and pulsatilla. However, each homeopathic medicine is designed to treat a very specific set of symptoms, so talk to a healthcare provider who can advise you on the best homeopathic for your situation.

- Drink cranberry juice and eat cranberries! Some types of heartburn can be caused by the bacteria H. *pylori*. Eating cranberries can potentially prevent this bacteria from attaching to your stomach lining, which helps to reduce heartburn.

- Acupuncture and acupressure treatment can balance the spleen and stomach if these organs are the cause of your heartburn.

- Sometimes heartburn is caused because of a lack of digestive acids being produced to break down food effectively. Adding lemon juice, a couple drops of essential oil of lemon or mandarin, or a teaspoon of apple cider vinegar to fresh water to drink after meals can help balance the acidity in the stomach.

- Often pregnant women experience rebound heartburn when taking products that include calcium carbonate, a commonly prescribed treatment for heartburn. These products do such a good job at destroying acid that the stomach has to overproduce acid just to digest its next meal. Often heartburn is related to too little acid, not too much.

Restless Legs: This annoying syndrome is common in pregnancy due to the prevalence of both anemia (low iron) and hypoglycemia (low blood sugar). Both of these conditions can increase the risk of Restless Legs Syndrome. Symptoms include an inability to relax your legs and/or a feeling that a current of electricity is running up and down your legs. Your legs can also feel shaky and jittery.

- Get your iron levels checked. If you are anemic, you can try eating iron-rich foods or taking the supplement Floradix to increase iron naturally.
- Make sure to eat several small meals a day and don't go long periods of time without eating to avoid drops in your blood sugar.
- Check your whole food vitamins and make certain they contain enough folic acid (400-800ug/mcg) and vitamin E (300iu), both important in reducing symptoms of Restless Leg Syndrome.
- Take a warm bath filled with Epsom salts before bed.

Stretch Marks: As your body expands due to your pregnancy, your skin can be stressed and leave stretch marks. Though there is not much that can be done to avoid stretch marks, you can keep your body hydrated and well nourished to keep the elasticity in your skin at an optimal level. It can also be helpful to keep your skin moisturized to keep the tissue flexible and avoid itchiness and scratching, which can exacerbate stretch marks. Once they appear, no cream will help make them disappear. Stretch marks do tend to get lighter and fade with time.

- Focus on eating foods rich in zinc such as sesame seeds, peanuts, pumpkin seeds, and dark chocolate. Vitamin C and vitamin E are also important components for nourished skin. It is also helpful to eat foods high in essential fatty acid and silica, a mineral that is essential for healthy skin. Silica can be found in abundance in celery.

- Cocoa butter can be used to moisturize your skin in areas where stretch marks tend to occur. While cocoa butter cannot prevent stretch marks from occurring, it can minimize the appearance and keep your skin from being itchy due to dryness.

- Essential oils that tend to be used in treatment of stretch marks are lavender, myrrh, frankincense, mandarin, and geranium. If you wish to use these essential oils, mix them into a carrier oil such as grapeseed oil, jojoba oil, or sweet almond oil. It is recommended that essential oils not be applied directly on the skin but instead mixed with a carrier oil to prevent skin irritation. You can massage areas affected by stretch marks with the essential oil mixture several times a day.

Nature Knows Best

For the majority of mothers, pregnancy naturally lasts between 37 and 42 weeks. When your baby is ready to be born, her lungs will have matured, her brain will have reached significant milestones of development, and the rest of her organ systems will be ready for life outside the womb. Contrary to popular belief, no one can tell you when your due date is. In fact, when people refer to the "due date" they leave off the most important word, estimated, for "estimated due date." Your pregnancy will last as long as your baby needs it to, based on your genetics, your nutrition, and your baby's individual needs. Every baby is different.

However, there are some situations when labor may start before your baby is fully developed. This is called pre-term labor, and occurs anytime that labor starts before 37 weeks of pregnancy. While all of the causes of preterm labor are not known, there are certain conditions and or situations that increase the risk of having a preterm labor:

- High levels of unresolved stress in the mother
- Elevated blood pressure or pre-eclampsia
- Being pregnant with more than one baby, such as twins or triplets
- Drug or alcohol use during pregnancy
- Obesity or being severely underweight
- Uterine or cervical abnormality
- Infections of the urinary tract or vagina
- Sexually transmitted diseases
- Blood clotting disorders

If you experience any one or more of the following symptoms prior to 37 weeks pregnant contact your healthcare provider:

- More than four uterine contractions in an hour: Uterine contractions are when the uterus tightens and becomes hard in an effort to move your baby down the birth canal. Make note: These contractions are different than Braxton-Hicks contractions, which normally occur during the last weeks of pregnancy. Braxton-Hicks contractions are infrequent, have no consistent pattern, and prepare the uterus for labor.
- Menstrual-like cramps: These cramps, which can sometimes be uterine contractions, may come and go or feel like constant cramping. Occasionally cramping occurs with diarrhea.
- Low, dull backache: This backache may move to the side of your waist or to your lower abdomen.
- Contractions that do not go away after drinking enough water to hydrate yourself.
- Contractions that do not go away after changing position.
- Pelvic pressure: Pressure in your pelvic area, low back or thighs.
- Leaking fluid or blood from your vagina. The fluid may

be watery or mucous-like and could be pink, light brown, or green.

- You have a feeling that "something isn't right."

Note about inductions: While you may be tempted to ask your care provider to induce your labor prior to 42 weeks, this may not be in you or your baby's best interest. Induction can lead to the birth of a preterm infant and/or increase your risk of medical intervention and cesarean. In the event that the topic of induction does come up, make sure to have an in-depth conversation with your healthcare provider and use conscious agreement to make the decision that is best for you and your baby.

Prenatal and Postpartum Mood and Anxiety Disorders (PMAD)

Mood and anxiety disorders during pregnancy and the postpartum period are on the rise. It's no surprise considering the fast-paced, high-stress lifestyle of today's society, coupled with the added demands of becoming a parent. While you may have heard of postpartum depression, very little media attention has been given to depression *during* pregnancy. Often postpartum mood and anxiety disorders (PMAD) begin during pregnancy. Prenatally, these disorders can include depression and anxiety, obsessive-compulsive disorder, panic disorder, and bipolar disorder. In fact, there are estimates that between 15 to 23 percent of pregnant women suffer from depression. When the symptoms of PMAD during pregnancy are ignored and not treated, the risks for increased symptoms during the postpartum period are higher.

The symptoms of PMAD prenatally can often be mistaken for common symptoms of pregnancy such as insomnia, exhaustion, inability to focus (pregnancy brain), anxiety, worry, and fatigue. Additional symptoms that may indicate PMAD include a decrease in appetite, lack of joy, guilt, feelings of hopelessness, and an inability to feel refreshed after resting. If you experience any symptoms of PMAD, taking a proactive approach can help you navigate through this short period in your life safely. Taking care of yourself prenatally and getting the treatment you need for PMAD can help reduce the risk of increased symptoms once your baby arrives.

Physical risk factors for developing PMAD include:
- History of depression
- Family history of mental illness
- Premenstrual dysphoria disorder
- Thyroid illness
- Very long or very short intervals between pregnancies
- Undergoing fertility treatments

Emotional risk factors include:
- Unsupportive or uninvolved spouse or partner
- Poor relationship with your own mother
- Feelings of ambivalence about becoming a mother
- Past emotional trauma
- Chemical dependency issues for anyone in the family
- Previous unresolved losses (such as abortion, miscarriage, stillbirth)

What to do:
If you are experiencing any of these symptoms, understand that PMAD is a real illness, and like any other illness, treatment and support are important for recovery. Often mothers feel a sense of guilt or shame when they are experiencing the symptoms of PMAD and are hesitant to contact their healthcare provider or reach out to anyone. Understand that you are not alone, many women experience PMAD as a result of the hormones associated with pregnancy and postpartum. PMAD does resolve with treatment. Common treatments include:

Phototherapy: This treatment exposes you to specific wavelengths of light that help regulate hormone production.

Blue blocking light therapy: This treatment involves wearing glasses that help to block blue light. Limiting blue light can help increase the brain's production of melatonin, which helps regulate sleep. Productive sleep helps regulate hormone production.

Nutritional therapy: This often includes specialized diets that are high in protein and essential fatty acids. Additionally, many therapists suggest the use of broad-spectrum micronutrient nutritional supplements.

Antidepressant medication: Some women respond very well to medication to control anxiety and depression. There are medications that are considered safe for use during pregnancy and while breastfeeding.

There are many resources for women experiencing PMAD. As a first step, talk to your healthcare provider openly and honestly about how you are feeling. Specifically ask for a referral to a good therapist who can identify the best treatments for your symptoms. Don't assume your partner recognizes or understands the symptoms of PMAD. Partners need resources and information so they can be a part of your support team. Both you and your partner can find online support groups and resources. Two excellent books to help you better understand PMAD are Beyond the Blues: A Guide to Understanding and Treating Prenatal and Postpartum Depression by Shoshana S. Bennett and Pec Indman and Transition to Parenthood: Myths, Reality and What Really Matters by Diana Lynn Barnes, Leigh G. Balber, Roberta Michnick Golinkoff, and Kathy Hirsh-Pasek.

Chapter 18

Nutrition in the Third Trimester

There is fascinating new evidence that your placenta communicates with your brain to help direct the development of your baby. Your placenta produces serotonin, which helps aid in the development of your baby's pancreas, brain, and heart. If your diet is not rich in the foods that help with seratonin production, your baby's development can be hindered. An important essential amino acid for seratonin development is tryptophan, which should be plentiful in your diet during your pregnancy. Some excellent sources of tryptophan are egg whites, chocolate, oats, dried dates, milk and yogurt, animal proteins, pumpkin seeds, and peanuts.

During the third trimester, your baby begins to develop her palate, or develop her "taste" for certain foods. The flavor oils of the foods you eat enter the amniotic fluid, which your baby can taste. What you eat affects your baby's future appetite. Research indicates that babies who are exposed to high levels of sugar, fat, and salt in the womb develop different reward centers in their brains. This means they become more likely as children and later on as adults to crave these unhealthy foods, which can increase their risk for obesity and other diseases. An unhealthy diet during pregnancy can contribute to the development of diabetes and heart disease later in your child's life. There is also evidence that eating foods that protect you from cancer-causing chemicals can also decrease your baby's risk of cancer later on. These are foods like cruciferous vegetables (broccoli and cauliflower) and green tea. You can create a healthy appetite and impact your baby's long-term health by consuming healthy and nutritious foods during the third trimester.

It becomes very important to focus on eating a rainbow of foods during this trimester, not only to ensure that you are nourishing your body and your growing baby, but also to help your baby learn to love a wide variety of flavors and foods. You are your child's first teacher, even in utero. Teach her to love healthy foods and unique, nutritious flavors. It might be fun to try a new food every day. Try vegetables you have never tasted before. Sample fruits from around the world. Try ethnic foods that you have never tasted before. Most importantly, eat the healthy foods that your family normally loves to eat in abundance to help your child develop a taste for them. This will help you avoid the pitfall of having to make two meals at every sitting, one for the adults and one for the children.

Due to the fact that your expanding uterus and growing baby have taken up a great deal of space in your body, your digestive system literally has a lot of pressure on it. Ensuring that every meal has healthy fiber options can keep things moving! A diet high in fiber can prevent constipation. Examples of good fiber options include black beans, whole fruits and vegetables, nuts, and seeds.

There is also growing evidence that a diet rich with essential fatty acids can help reduce the risk of preeclampsia. Preeclampsia is a condition that is associated with the following symptoms: headache, blurry vision, sudden swelling and weight gain, high blood pressure, and protein in the urine. It is a dangerous condition and must be treated immediately. The only true solution to this illness is giving birth. It is not something that can go untreated because the condition can cause damage to the mother's kidneys and reduce the blood flow available to the placenta. There is some evidence that high stress levels increase the risk of preeclampsia, and by now you should know how to help yourself manage stress. Additionally, there are some nutritional considerations to help with prevention. Low protein levels have long been associated with increased risk of preeclampsia. Getting enough protein is important not only for this reason, but also because your baby is experiencing rapid growth during this time and protein helps provide the amino acids necessary for this job.

During the third trimester it is important to focus on foods rich in essential fatty acids. Of particular significance is the omega-3 fatty acid, DHA. Your baby's brain is growing by leaps and bounds during this trimester. In the last few weeks, her brain doubles in size and matures significantly. That means the neural connections in your baby's brain are occurring at incredibly fast rates. Her brain is primarily made of fat, and therefore needs essential fatty acids to grow correctly. An excellent source of DHA is wild caught salmon. Studies show that moms who consumed more fish during pregnancy (at least four servings a week) had babies with higher cognitive developmental scores. Evening primrose oil (EPO) is another excellent source of essential fatty acids. EPO helps your body to produce prostaglandins, which are necessary for healthy digestion, fluid regulation, healthy blood pressure, and pain management. Prostaglandins are also necessary to help your cervix become soft and supple to dilate effectively during labor. Some studies also show that supplementing with EPO can reduce the risk of preeclampsia.

Fish oil supplements can also be surprisingly beneficial for you during this trimester. They are rich with essential fatty acids that can not only help with your baby's brain growth, but they can also help with the prevention and management of pregnancy, and postpartum mood and anxiety disorders. If you are not getting enough essential fatty acids in your diet, it can lead to mood imbalances and foggy thinking. Supplementing your diet with healthy fish oils can reduce this risk, especially if you do not eat enough fish in your everyday diet. Studies have shown that ingesting fish oil can help reduce the risk of preterm labor and is associated with healthier weights in newborns. Try taking a supplement every day that includes at least one gram of fish oil (though up to six grams during pregnancy is still considered safe). Some fish oils have added citrus to improve aftertaste. Check with your healthcare provider for the correct dosage.

Ultimately your body is a reflection of your emotional health. When you love yourself by honoring your feelings, taking care, and nourishing yourself, you can have the greatest pregnancy ever.

🗝 Honor the third trimester as a time of nesting and preparation by having a blessingway performed for you.

🗝 Create a vision board as a map towards a great birth experience.

🗝 Perceptions of Pain

- The pain of labor is a sign your body is working for you.
- Contractions are intermittent in labor and you have plenty of time to rest in between.
- There are many natural options for pain management.
- Labor intensifies slowly so your body has time to adjust.
- Vocalization is normal and helpful for labor.

🗝 Optimal fetal positioning is a technique you can use in the last weeks of pregnancy to help your baby line up for an easier, quicker, and more comfortable labor.

🗝 Create your best labor nest

- Decide now who will be with you during your labor.
- Use a birth plan as a tool for clarifying your belief systems, but rely on your communication skills and your birth team during labor to have the birth you want.

- Consider creating a vision board instead of, or in addition to, a birth plan.
- Have open and honest communication with your healthcare providers during pregnancy. Don't wait to share your thoughts until you are in labor.
- Carefully select your healthcare team and place of birth early in pregnancy.
- Use conscious agreement for any and all healthcare decisions.

Take time prenatally to discuss your feelings with your partner about the following decisions that impact the health of your baby: breastfeeding, practicing skin-to-skin, common newborn procedures (such as antibiotic eye ointment), circumcision, vaccines and immunizations, and choosing a pediatrician for your baby.

Make plans during your last trimester for life after pregnancy. Things to consider include:

- Prepare for nourishment for you and your partner in the early days and weeks postpartum.
- Plan to have a "babymoon" in the early days postpartum.
- Communicate your boundaries to your family and friends.
- Make a plan for housework after the baby arrives.
- Create the ideal nest in one or two rooms where you will spend the most time with your baby. Stock up on the items you will need and arrange the room so it is comfortable for you.
- Arrange for postpartum help ahead of time.
- Consider any siblings and make plans to help ease the transition to big brother or sister.

- Make plans to ease the transition for your pets and have strategies in place for pet safety in your home for your baby.

🗝 Interview your place of birth early in your pregnancy. Decide whether you want a homebirth, birth center birth, or hospital birth.

🗝 Consider hiring a doula.

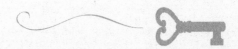

Final Thoughts

While you may have come to the end of this book, you are really at a beginning. It's the beginning of a new you, a new family, and one of the most profound relationships you will ever have. Becoming a mother is a journey that will bring you the greatest love you will ever experience, while also experiencing incredible joy, pain, and sorrow. Your children will present you with the lessons of a lifetime. They will teach you patience and compassion and will push you to the very edge of sanity. All the while, you will be astonished by the very depth of your love for them. You will learn that you are stronger than you ever knew you could be. There will be mistakes made along the journey. Life is messy, it's juicy, it's joyful, it's terrifying, and it's supposed to be that way. Out of the chaos comes beauty, and this is the lesson of mothering.

While this book has given you keys to help guide you through your pregnancy, we hope that you remember that you already have the master key inside yourself. You have every parenting answer you will ever need. When you need answers, remember conscious agreement, listen carefully to your inner wisdom, and trust yourself.

You are about to meet the love of your life. We wish you love, laughter, joy, and strength along your journey. Ultimately, we wish you *the greatest pregnancy ever!*

Love and light,
Tracy and Laurel

The Beginning...

About the Authors

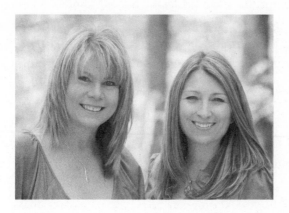

Tracy and Laurel wrote the *Greatest Pregnancy Ever* with the hope to unite evidence-based information with heart and mind science to give parents the tools they need to feel deeply bonded to their pregnancy and their baby.

Tracy Wilson Peters, CLD, CLE, CCCE, has been a lifelong advocate for families and babies. Married for over 19 years and mother to two amazing sons, Tracy's experience raising her own children led her to a love for supporting expectant families. This passion encouraged her to found CAPPA, Childbirth and Postpartum Professionals Association. Tracy serves as both the CEO and as a faculty member for CAPPA. CAPPA is the largest childbirth organization in the world. Internationally known as a pregnancy expert, she has authored numerous articles, and appeared on many television networks, including FOX, CBS, and NBC. Tracy has worked with expectant women and families for nearly two decades, attending hundreds of births as a professional labor doula and teaching classes to more than 3000 families.

Laurel Wilson, IBCLC, CLE, CCCE, CLD, has over sixteen years of experience working with families and professionals as a childbirth and lactation educator/trainer, doula, lactation consultant, and prenatal yoga instructor. Laurel takes a creative approach to working with the pregnant family, helping families to connect with their inner resources to discover their true beliefs about themselves, their relationships, and their abilities to birth and parent their children. Laurel has successfully trained hundreds of professionals to become childbirth and lactation educators, labor doulas, and prenatal yoga teachers. She has been featured as a pregnancy and breastfeeding expert in professional videos and webinars. Laurel has been joyfully married to her husband for 20 years and has two beautiful sons, whose difficult births led her on a path towards helping emerging families create positive experiences. She believes that the journey into parenthood is a life-changing rite of passage that should be deeply honored and celebrated.

Look for Tracy and Laurel's upcoming books from Lotus Life Press:
Manifest Your Birth
Keys To The MotherBaby Bond: Postpartum and Breastfeeding

For inquiries on speaking engagements, lectures and book signings, please email info@thegreatestpregnancyever.com.

Connect With Us
You can find more information on the concepts in this book, current research and resources by visiting the following sites:

www.thegreatestpregnancyever.com
www.facebook.com/thegreatestpregnancyever
www.twitter.com/great_pregnancy
info@thegreatestpregnancyever.com

Index